THE COMPLETE RUNNER'S DAY-BY-DAY LOG 2024 CALENDAR

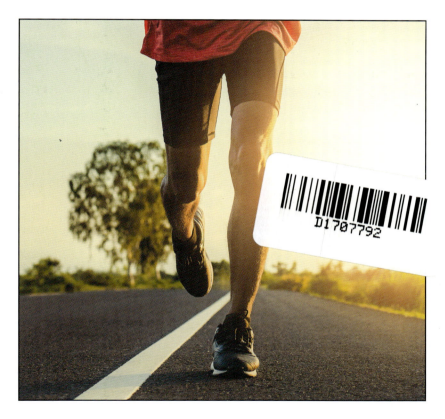

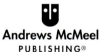

Andrews McMeel
PUBLISHING®

MATT FITZGERALD
Author of *On Pace*, Cofounder of 80/20 Endurance

2023

January
S	M	T	W	T	F	S
1	2	3	4	5	6	7
8	9	10	11	12	13	14
15	16	17	18	19	20	21
22	23	24	25	26	27	28
29	30	31				

February
S	M	T	W	T	F	S
			1	2	3	4
5	6	7	8	9	10	11
12	13	14	15	16	17	18
19	20	21	22	23	24	25
26	27	28				

March
S	M	T	W	T	F	S
			1	2	3	4
5	6	7	8	9	10	11
12	13	14	15	16	17	18
19	20	21	22	23	24	25
26	27	28	29	30	31	

April
S	M	T	W	T	F	S
						1
2	3	4	5	6	7	8
9	10	11	12	13	14	15
16	17	18	19	20	21	22
23	24	25	26	27	28	29
30						

May
S	M	T	W	T	F	S
	1	2	3	4	5	6
7	8	9	10	11	12	13
14	15	16	17	18	19	20
21	22	23	24	25	26	27
28	29	30	31			

June
S	M	T	W	T	F	S
				1	2	3
4	5	6	7	8	9	10
11	12	13	14	15	16	17
18	19	20	21	22	23	24
25	26	27	28	29	30	

July
S	M	T	W	T	F	S
						1
2	3	4	5	6	7	8
9	10	11	12	13	14	15
16	17	18	19	20	21	22
23	24	25	26	27	28	29
30	31					

August
S	M	T	W	T	F	S
		1	2	3	4	5
6	7	8	9	10	11	12
13	14	15	16	17	18	19
20	21	22	23	24	25	26
27	28	29	30	31		

September
S	M	T	W	T	F	S
					1	2
3	4	5	6	7	8	9
10	11	12	13	14	15	16
17	18	19	20	21	22	23
24	25	26	27	28	29	30

October
S	M	T	W	T	F	S
1	2	3	4	5	6	7
8	9	10	11	12	13	14
15	16	17	18	19	20	21
22	23	24	25	26	27	28
29	30	31				

November
S	M	T	W	T	F	S
			1	2	3	4
5	6	7	8	9	10	11
12	13	14	15	16	17	18
19	20	21	22	23	24	25
26	27	28	29	30		

December
S	M	T	W	T	F	S
					1	2
3	4	5	6	7	8	9
10	11	12	13	14	15	16
17	18	19	20	21	22	23
24	25	26	27	28	29	30
31						

2025

January
S	M	T	W	T	F	S
			1	2	3	4
5	6	7	8	9	10	11
12	13	14	15	16	17	18
19	20	21	22	23	24	25
26	27	28	29	30	31	

February
S	M	T	W	T	F	S
						1
2	3	4	5	6	7	8
9	10	11	12	13	14	15
16	17	18	19	20	21	22
23	24	25	26	27	28	

March
S	M	T	W	T	F	S
						1
2	3	4	5	6	7	8
9	10	11	12	13	14	15
16	17	18	19	20	21	22
23	24	25	26	27	28	29
30	31					

April
S	M	T	W	T	F	S
		1	2	3	4	5
6	7	8	9	10	11	12
13	14	15	16	17	18	19
20	21	22	23	24	25	26
27	28	29	30			

May
S	M	T	W	T	F	S
				1	2	3
4	5	6	7	8	9	10
11	12	13	14	15	16	17
18	19	20	21	22	23	24
25	26	27	28	29	30	31

June
S	M	T	W	T	F	S
1	2	3	4	5	6	7
8	9	10	11	12	13	14
15	16	17	18	19	20	21
22	23	24	25	26	27	28
29	30					

July
S	M	T	W	T	F	S
		1	2	3	4	5
6	7	8	9	10	11	12
13	14	15	16	17	18	19
20	21	22	23	24	25	26
27	28	29	30	31		

August
S	M	T	W	T	F	S
					1	2
3	4	5	6	7	8	9
10	11	12	13	14	15	16
17	18	19	20	21	22	23
24	25	26	27	28	29	30
31						

September
S	M	T	W	T	F	S
	1	2	3	4	5	6
7	8	9	10	11	12	13
14	15	16	17	18	19	20
21	22	23	24	25	26	27
28	29	30				

October
S	M	T	W	T	F	S
			1	2	3	4
5	6	7	8	9	10	11
12	13	14	15	16	17	18
19	20	21	22	23	24	25
26	27	28	29	30	31	

November
S	M	T	W	T	F	S
						1
2	3	4	5	6	7	8
9	10	11	12	13	14	15
16	17	18	19	20	21	22
23	24	25	26	27	28	29
30						

December
S	M	T	W	T	F	S
	1	2	3	4	5	6
7	8	9	10	11	12	13
14	15	16	17	18	19	20
21	22	23	24	25	26	27
28	29	30	31			

2024

January
S	M	T	W	T	F	S
	1	2	3	4	5	6
7	8	9	10	11	12	13
14	15	16	17	18	19	20
21	22	23	24	25	26	27
28	29	30	31			

February
S	M	T	W	T	F	S
				1	2	3
4	5	6	7	8	9	10
11	12	13	14	15	16	17
18	19	20	21	22	23	24
25	26	27	28	29		

March
S	M	T	W	T	F	S
					1	2
3	4	5	6	7	8	9
10	11	12	13	14	15	16
17	18	19	20	21	22	23
24	25	26	27	28	29	30
31						

April
S	M	T	W	T	F	S
	1	2	3	4	5	6
7	8	9	10	11	12	13
14	15	16	17	18	19	20
21	22	23	24	25	26	27
28	29	30				

May
S	M	T	W	T	F	S
			1	2	3	4
5	6	7	8	9	10	11
12	13	14	15	16	17	18
19	20	21	22	23	24	25
26	27	28	29	30	31	

June
S	M	T	W	T	F	S
						1
2	3	4	5	6	7	8
9	10	11	12	13	14	15
16	17	18	19	20	21	22
23	24	25	26	27	28	29
30						

July
S	M	T	W	T	F	S
	1	2	3	4	5	6
7	8	9	10	11	12	13
14	15	16	17	18	19	20
21	22	23	24	25	26	27
28	29	30	31			

August
S	M	T	W	T	F	S
				1	2	3
4	5	6	7	8	9	10
11	12	13	14	15	16	17
18	19	20	21	22	23	24
25	26	27	28	29	30	31

September
S	M	T	W	T	F	S
1	2	3	4	5	6	7
8	9	10	11	12	13	14
15	16	17	18	19	20	21
22	23	24	25	26	27	28
29	30					

October
S	M	T	W	T	F	S
		1	2	3	4	5
6	7	8	9	10	11	12
13	14	15	16	17	18	19
20	21	22	23	24	25	26
27	28	29	30	31		

November
S	M	T	W	T	F	S
					1	2
3	4	5	6	7	8	9
10	11	12	13	14	15	16
17	18	19	20	21	22	23
24	25	26	27	28	29	30

December
S	M	T	W	T	F	S
1	2	3	4	5	6	7
8	9	10	11	12	13	14
15	16	17	18	19	20	21
22	23	24	25	26	27	28
29	30	31				

INTRODUCTION

On Christmas Day 1986, my parents gave me a brand-new, spiral-bound running log, a daily planner with a male runner's lean, striding legs on the front cover. It wasn't the costliest gift I found under the tree that year, but it was the most valuable.

Fifteen at the time, I'd already been running for a few years but had committed to the sport more recently, after blowing out my knee playing soccer. Over the next twelve months I recorded the basic facts of every workout and race I completed as a member of the Oyster River High School track and cross-country teams (Go, Bobcats!). Day by day, what began as an ordered stack of mostly empty pages transformed into the story of a boy falling irreversibly in love with running.

Thirty-five years later, I received the same gift a second time—sort of. It came in the form of an email message from an editor with Andrews McMeel Publishing, inviting me to become the new author of *The Complete Runner's Day-by-Day Log*—the same planner I'd used as a kid. My father, who got me into running, likes to say that "circles are the only geometry in life," a truth we runners understand better than anyone. No matter how far we go, we always seem to end up where we started, albeit changed.

Naturally, I leapt at this opportunity. Certain events have a way of pinching the soul with a keen sense of time's irreversible passage, making long-ago bits of our lives seem both palpably immediate and galactically remote, and this project, for me, was one of them. Also, calendars are all about time. And so is running.

To become a runner is to experience time differently. In a world of instant gratification, running cultivates the acquired taste of delayed gratification, demanding and rewarding patience, and thereby teaching this timeless virtue. As runners we take the long view, like those medieval cathedral builders who toiled on structures they would never see completed; we prize the journey above the destination. Indeed, the destination is just an excuse for the journey.

Time changes when we run. During easy jogs our minds wander as our brains enter a state that neuroscientists refer to, somewhat opaquely, as default network activation. When we snap back to the present, we're miles down the road, wondering how we got there. In harder workouts we sometimes enter a flow state, where time slows as we seem to become the very act of running. And in races, it often feels as if we experience an entire lifetime in the span of a few hours or less. So much can happen in 26.2 miles!

I served as a coach at a running camp with a colleague of mine who comes from a swimming background. Afterward she expressed surprise at how fixated the attendees were on time, particularly on improving their personal bests for various race distances. It all seemed rather superficial to her, a self-imposed barrier to a deeper experience of running—but we know better. By focusing on time, we test our limits, and by testing our limits we in fact experience a richer, more transformative journey than we would if we didn't count the seconds—or keep meticulous running logs.

Another way in which running functions as a kind of time travel has to do with its primal ancientness. Millions of years ago, when our primate ancestors came down from the trees, they did not know how to run. But their descendants learned, and in so doing, they became human.

I can feel this history in my body when I run, and I'll bet you can, too. The older I get, the more I think of today's runners, myself included, as temporary stewards of a great tradition given to us by past generations, one that we will pass on—a beautiful and never-ending torch relay.

It's in this spirit that I assume authorship of *The Complete Runner's Day-by-Day Log*. Started by the legendary James F. Fixx (those were his legs on the cover of my 1987 copy), this venerable tradition-within-a-tradition was handed down to John Jerome, a terrific writer who in turn handed it down to his son, the equally terrific Marty Jerome. Now it's my turn, and I intend to make the most of it, honoring the legacy I've inherited to the very best of my ability, until it's time to pass the torch.

—Matt Fitzgerald ■

January

SUNDAY	MONDAY	TUESDAY	WEDNESDAY	THURSDAY	FRIDAY	SATURDAY
	1 New Year's Day Kwanzaa ends (USA)	2 New Year's Day (observed) (NZ, UK–Scotland)	3	4 ◐ Last Quarter	5	6
7	8	9	10	11 ● New Moon	12	13
14	15 Martin Luther King Jr. Day (USA)	16	17	18 ◐ First Quarter	19	20
21	22	23	24	25 ○ Full Moon	26 Australia Day	27
28	29	30	31			

tip: The purpose of setting goals is not to achieve them but to stretch you beyond present limits. Achieving a goal is nice, but any goal that moves you forward as a runner has done its job.

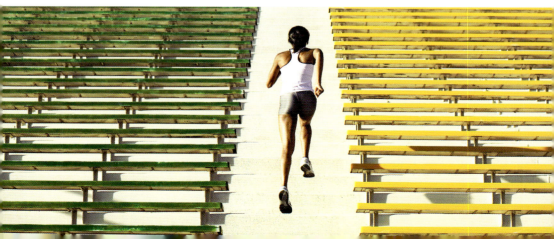

ALL IN THIS TOGETHER

I won a marathon once. It felt pretty good. But do you know what felt even better? The time I helped another runner win a marathon.

It was at a small event in eastern Virginia. I was just over five miles from finishing when I caught a runner who'd been ahead of me the entire race but was beginning to struggle. I made a spontaneous decision to slow down and run with her instead of surging ahead. I spoke words of encouragement, using her name—Kacey—after learning it from spectators, and I even stopped when she stopped to stretch out a cramping hamstring. When she pulled up a second time, with less than a mile to go, she waved me on, promising to meet me at the finish line. Only later, at the post-race awards ceremony, did I learn that Kacey had been leading the women's division when I caught her, and that, thanks in part to my assistance, she'd held on to win.

"You were my guardian angel out there," she told me.

Boy did that feel good! But why? I think it has something to do with human nature. Shared suffering forges human bonds like nothing else. Psychologists have demonstrated that people behave more altruistically after experiencing pain. Soldiers exhibit less severe symptoms of post-traumatic stress when deployed with their brothers-in-arms than when separated from them back home. Boxers embrace after the final bell puts an end to their efforts to flatten each other. Marathons and other running events transform strangers into comrades faster than you can say, "Golly, this sucks!"

My brief but intense encounter with Kacey recalled that well-known line of unknown origin, "Be kind, for everyone you meet is fighting a hard battle." No one would deny the wisdom of this counsel. In everyday life, though, it's easy to fail to see the hard battle others are fighting. But in a marathon, you can't miss it, and seeing your own suffering mirrored in others around you kindles solidarity that transcends the moment, creating an empathetic community which, for folks like Kacey and me—and probably you— makes running much more than a sport.

Technically, ours is an individual sport—every man and woman for himself or herself. But that's not how we really experience it, is it? We truly are all in this together and the experience is best for all of us when we remember this fact. ■

© Peter Griffith/gettyimages

Distance carried forward:

1 Monday 1

Where & When: **Distance:**
Comments:

2 Tuesday 2

Where & When: **Distance:**
Comments:

3 Wednesday 3

Where & When: **Distance:**
Comments:

4 Thursday 4

Where & When: **Distance:**
Comments:

5 Friday 5

Where & When: **Distance:**
Comments:

January

Saturday 6

Where & When: **Distance:**
Comments:

Sunday 7

Where & When: **Distance:**
Comments:

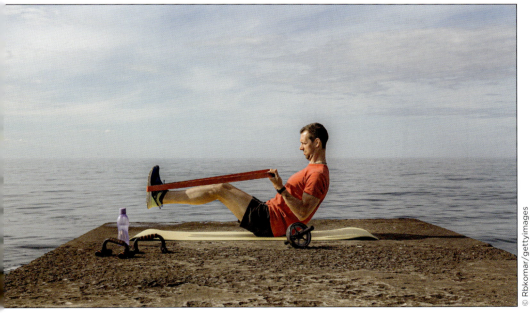

© Rbkomar/gettyimages

tip: To runners who feel they don't have time for strength training: Even two twenty-minute strength sessions per week are proven to reduce injury risk and improve running performance.

Distance this week: **Weight:**

Distance carried forward:

8 Monday

Where & When: **Distance:**
Comments:

9 Tuesday

Eliptical- 12min, .62 / mile

Where & When: **Distance:**
Comments:

10 Wednesday

Where & When: **Distance:**
Comments:

11 Thursday

Where & When: **Distance:**
Comments:

12 Friday

Where & When: **Distance:**
Comments:

January

Saturday 13

13

Where & When: Distance:
Comments:

Sunday 14

14

Where & When: Distance:
Comments:

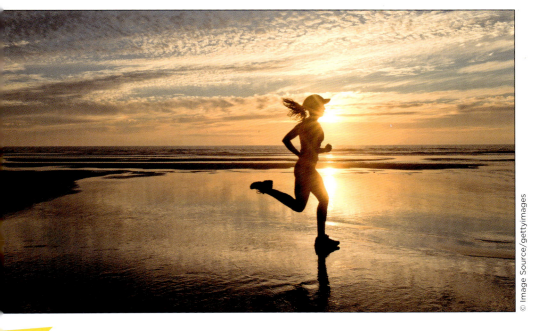

tip: In a recent study, the strongest psychological predictor of a successful ultramarathon finish was self-efficacy, or the belief in one's ability to succeed.

Distance this week: .62   Weight:

Distance carried forward:

15 Monday 15

Where & When: Distance:
Comments:

16 Tuesday 16

Where & When: Distance:
Comments:

17 Wednesday 17

Where & When: Distance:
Comments:

18 Thursday 18

Where & When: Distance:
Comments:

19 Friday 19

Where & When: Distance:
Comments:

January

Saturday 20

Where & When: Distance:

Comments:

Sunday 21

Where & When: Distance:

Comments:

© Jakob Helbig/gettyimages

tip: When Desiree Linden won the Boston Marathon in 2018 in atrocious weather, she credited her winter training in Michigan for toughening her up. You will be rewarded for getting out there and running!

Distance this week: Weight:

Distance carried forward: _____

22 Monday 22

_____
_____

Where & When: _____ **Distance:** _____
Comments: _____

23 Tuesday 23

_____
_____

Where & When: _____ **Distance:** _____
Comments: _____

24 Wednesday 24

_____
_____

Where & When: _____ **Distance:** _____
Comments: _____

25 Thursday 25

_____
_____

Where & When: _____ **Distance:** _____
Comments: _____

26 Friday 26

_____
_____

Where & When: _____ **Distance:** _____
Comments: _____

January

Saturday 27

27

Where & When: Distance:
Comments:

28 .50 x 2 = 1 mile **Sunday 28**

Where & When: Distance:
Comments:

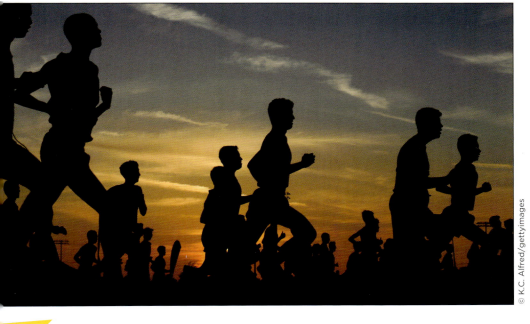

tip: If your training feels "too easy," that might be a good thing. Runners who make the mistake of doing all the training they can handle in the early part of the process tend to burn out later.

Distance this week: 1.0   Weight:

Distance carried forward: 1,62

29 Monday 29

Where & When: **Distance:**
Comments:

30 Tuesday 30

Where & When: **Distance:**
Comments:

31 Wednesday 31

Where & When: **Distance:**
Comments:

1 Thursday 32

Where & When: **Distance:**
Comments:

2 Friday 33

Where & When: **Distance:**
Comments:

Jan/Feb

Saturday 3

Where & When: Distance:
Comments:

Sunday 4

Where & When: Distance:
Comments:

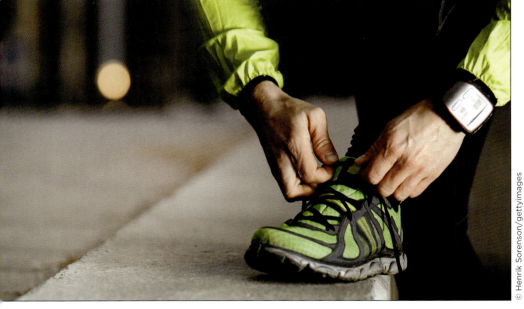

© Henrik Sorenson/gettyimages

tip: You get what you pay for with running gear. Don't settle for inferior products because you feel you're too slow or too new. Your running deserves the very best stuff that fits your budget!

Distance this week: Weight:

February

SUNDAY	MONDAY	TUESDAY	WEDNESDAY	THURSDAY	FRIDAY	SATURDAY
				1	2	3
					☽ Last Quarter	
4	5	6	7	8	9	10
	St. Brigid's Day (Ireland)	Waitangi Day (NZ)			● New Moon	Lunar New Year (Year of the Dragon)
11	12	13	14	15	16	17
			Ash Wednesday St. Valentine's Day		☽ First Quarter	
18	19	20	21	22	23	24
	Presidents' Day (USA)					○ Full Moon
25	26	27	28	29		

tip: If you tend to hit the wall in long runs, try the "fastest mile last" rule: The last mile of each long run must be your fastest, if only by a second or two. It forces you to think ahead, slowing down voluntarily early on instead of involuntarily later.

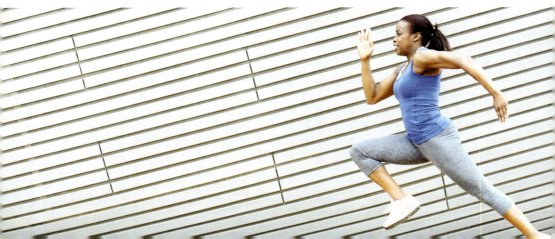

ASSUME NOTHING

I made certain assumptions as a younger runner. For example, I assumed that I would stop improving at age thirty-eight. This might sound like an arbitrary number, but in fact, no runner over thirty-eight held any existing world records at the time, so I figured if the best runners on the planet peaked by then, surely, I would, too.

As it turned out, I ran my fastest marathon at forty-six, and set a new personal-best time in the 10K three years later, on the cusp of turning fifty. Granted, it's not uncommon for runners to run their best races over forty, but those who do typically got a late start. I started running competitively at age eleven, completing my first 10K a year later. My marathon debut came at twenty-eight, and I had run forty more by the time I finally stopped getting faster, as every runner must eventually. (To my knowledge, no runner has ever set a personal-best race time after their two hundredth birthday.)

How did I defy my own expectations? There's no single answer. Taking care of my body—eating right, keeping fit, prioritizing sleep—was certainly one factor. Maintaining my passion for the sport was another. Elite runners (of which I was never one) who defy Father Time and remain on top past forty are invariably people whose enjoyment of running never fades. "I love running," said American runner Abdi Abdirahman before qualifying for his fifth Olympics at forty-three. "It's my hobby."

There's one other thing that factored into my surprisingly protracted running prime: At some point I stopped *expecting* to get slower with age and made no further assumptions about what was or wasn't possible in the future. This shift in mindset was inspired in part by Dave Scott, the legendary triathlete who won the Ironman World Championship six times before finishing second at age forty. When I asked Dave for the secret to his longevity, he answered that he simply refused to slow down. Others fade, he opined, because "they allow it."

Let me be clear: It's no sin to grow older, and we all slow down eventually. What's important is avoiding self-limiting expectations. My middle-aged running renaissance taught me a lesson that serves as a helpful motto, not just for me but for any runner: *Assume nothing!* ∎

Distance carried forward:

5 Monday 36

Where & When: Distance:
Comments:

6 Tuesday 37

Where & When: Distance:
Comments:

7 Wednesday 38

Where & When: Distance:
Comments:

8 Thursday 39

Where & When: Distance:
Comments:

9 Friday 40

Where & When: Distance:
Comments:

February

41
Saturday 10

Where & When: Distance:
Comments:

42
Sunday 11

Where & When: Distance:
Comments:

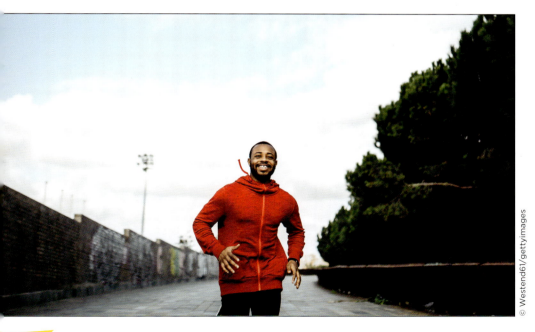

tip: Each runner responds differently to training. Some runners can handle a lot of miles, others can't handle a lot of speed work, and so on. Learn from your training and do more of what works for you and less of what doesn't.

Distance this week: Weight:

Distance carried forward: _____

12 Monday   43

_____
_____

Where & When: _____ **Distance:** _____
Comments: _____

13 Tuesday   44

_____
_____

Where & When: _____ **Distance:** _____
Comments: _____

14 Wednesday   45

_____
_____

Where & When: _____ **Distance:** _____
Comments: _____

15 Thursday   46

_____
_____

Where & When: _____ **Distance:** _____
Comments: _____

16 Friday   47

_____
_____

Where & When: _____ **Distance:** _____
Comments: _____

February

Saturday 17

Where & When: Distance:
Comments:

Sunday 18

Where & When: Distance:
Comments:

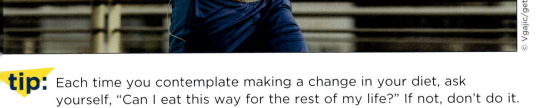

tip: Each time you contemplate making a change in your diet, ask yourself, "Can I eat this way for the rest of my life?" If not, don't do it.

Distance this week: Weight:

Distance carried forward: _____

19 Monday   50

_____
_____

Where & When: **Distance:**
Comments:

20 Tuesday   51

_____
_____

Where & When: **Distance:**
Comments:

21 Wednesday   52

_____
_____

Where & When: **Distance:**
Comments:

22 Thursday   53

_____
_____

Where & When: **Distance:**
Comments:

23 Friday   54

_____
_____

Where & When: **Distance:**
Comments:

February

55

Saturday 24

Where & When: Distance:
Comments:

56

Sunday 25

Where & When: Distance:
Comments:

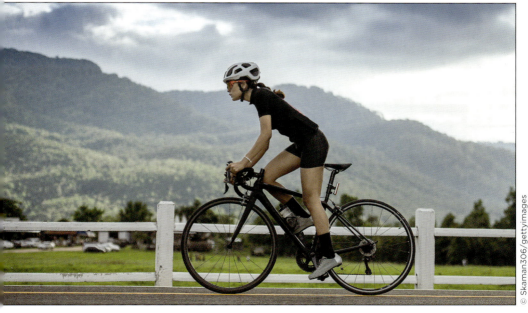

tip: Low-impact aerobic cross-training reduces injury risk and increases fitness in runners. The best cross-training activities approximate the running motion without the impact—bicycling, elliptical running, and incline treadmill walking.

Distance this week: Weight:

Distance carried forward: _____

26 Monday 57

_____
_____

Where & When: _____ **Distance:** _____
Comments: _____

27 Tuesday 58

_____
_____

Where & When: _____ **Distance:** _____
Comments: _____

28 Wednesday 59

_____
_____

Where & When: _____ **Distance:** _____
Comments: _____

29 Thursday 60

_____
_____

Where & When: _____ **Distance:** _____
Comments: _____

1 Friday 61

_____
_____

Where & When: _____ **Distance:** _____
Comments: _____

Feb/Mar

Saturday 2

Where & When: Distance:

Comments:

Sunday 3

Where & When: Distance:

Comments:

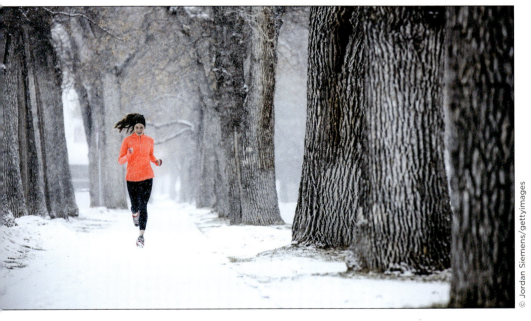

© Jordan Siemens/gettyimages

tip: If you've dressed properly for an outdoor run on a cold day, you should feel a little chilly when you start. This ensures you don't overheat later as your core body temperature rises.

Distance this week: Weight:

March

SUNDAY	MONDAY	TUESDAY	WEDNESDAY	THURSDAY	FRIDAY	SATURDAY
					1 St. David's Day (UK)	2
3 ☽ Last Quarter	4 Labour Day (Australia—WA)	5	6	7	8 International Women's Day	9
10 ● New Moon Ramadan Daylight Saving Time begins (USA, Canada) Mothering Sunday (Ireland, UK)	11 Eight Hours Day (Australia—TAS) Labour Day (Australia—VIC) Commonwealth Day (Australia, Canada, NZ, UK)	12	13	14	15	16
17 ☾ First Quarter St. Patrick's Day	18	19	20 Vernal Equinox	21	22	23 Purim (begins at sundown)
24 Palm Sunday	25	26	27	28	29 Good Friday (Western)	30
31 Easter (Western)	○ Full Moon					

tip: Before important races, take some time to close your eyes and visualize the process of making your way through the course. Try to make these mental rehearsals as realistic as possible. Imagine a challenging but ultimately successful experience.

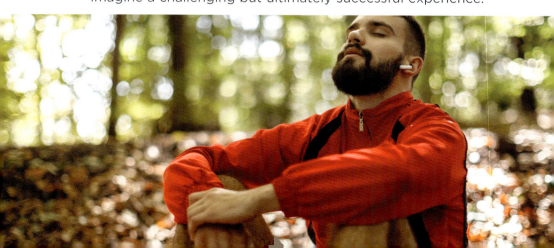

FEELING GOOD

I used to coach an athlete who went to the Olympics in Greco-Roman wrestling. To be clear, I coached her for running, not wrestling, but you knew that.

I'd been working with Jessie for a few weeks when she asked me if I thought she was training hard enough. "I do," I said. "Why do you ask?"

"Because I feel really good!" Jessie explained that, throughout her wrestling career, she and her fellow elite wrestlers trained hard all the time, so she got used to feeling kind of lousy. In fact, feeling lousy became something she thought of as indicating that she was training properly, which was why she wondered if she was working hard enough with me. I have no idea if wrestlers are supposed to train so hard they feel lousy, but I do know that runners *should feel good* most of the time and should modulate their training in ways that minimize the amount of time they feel lousy.

This statement seems counterintuitive to a lot of runners, and not just those who were previously world-class wrestlers. Whenever I encounter such a runner, I tell them about Eliud Kipchoge, who is widely regarded as the greatest marathoner in history. In a book about him, authors Tait Hearps and Matt Inglis Fox expressed surprise at how restrained the Kenyan legend was during his training for the 2017 Berlin Marathon, writing, "Eliud seldom seemed to reach a point where he was maximally exerted. I can't recall a grimace on his face during a workout. He and the other athletes worked very hard; however, they methodically trained in a way that gradually built fitness, refraining from all-out efforts, and retaining reserves of energy for the most critical of exertions, when it mattered most."

Understand that a runner must train fairly hard to feel good most of the time. That's because it feels good to be fit, and you need to train fairly hard to get fit. The thing to avoid is training so hard that you're in a continuous state of fatigue, which does not feel good. I can't speak for you, but for me, the fact that feeling good most of the time is a sure sign you're training properly is one more reason to love running! ■

Distance carried forward:

4 Monday 64

Where & When: **Distance:**
Comments:

5 Tuesday 65

Where & When: **Distance:**
Comments:

6 Wednesday 66

Where & When: **Distance:**
Comments:

7 Thursday 67

Where & When: **Distance:**
Comments:

8 Friday 68

Where & When: **Distance:**
Comments:

March

Saturday 9

Where & When:　　　　　　　　　　　　Distance:
Comments:

Sunday 10

Where & When:　　　　　　　　　　　　Distance:
Comments:

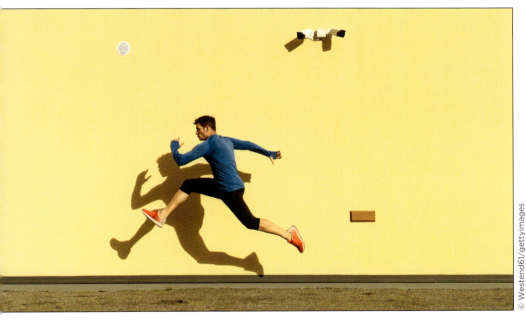

tip: Contrary to popular belief, a stride rate of one hundred and eighty steps per minute is not optimal for all runners. Your cadence will self-optimize over time if you just keep running and don't think about it.

Distance this week:　　　　　　　　　　Weight:

Distance carried forward: _____

11 Monday   71

_____
_____

Where & When: _____ **Distance:** _____
Comments: _____

12 Tuesday   72

_____
_____

Where & When: _____ **Distance:** _____
Comments: _____

13 Wednesday   73

_____
_____

Where & When: _____ **Distance:** _____
Comments: _____

14 Thursday   74

_____
_____

Where & When: _____ **Distance:** _____
Comments: _____

15 Friday   75

_____
_____

Where & When: _____ **Distance:** _____
Comments: _____

March

Saturday 16

Where & When: Distance:
Comments:

Sunday 17

Where & When: Distance:
Comments:

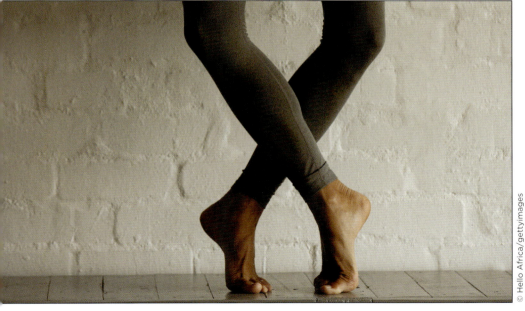

tip: Foot-strengthening exercises such as big-toe lifts are proven to reduce injury risk in runners. Don't neglect this important part of your body in your strength routine!

Distance this week: Weight:

Distance carried forward:

18 Monday 78

Where & When: **Distance:**
Comments:

19 Tuesday 79

Where & When: **Distance:**
Comments:

20 Wednesday 80

Where & When: **Distance:**
Comments:

21 Thursday 81

Where & When: **Distance:**
Comments:

22 Friday 82

Where & When: **Distance:**
Comments:

March

Saturday 23
83

Where & When: **Distance:**
Comments:

Sunday 24
84

Rivermalk Area

Where & When: **Distance:** 1 mile
Comments:

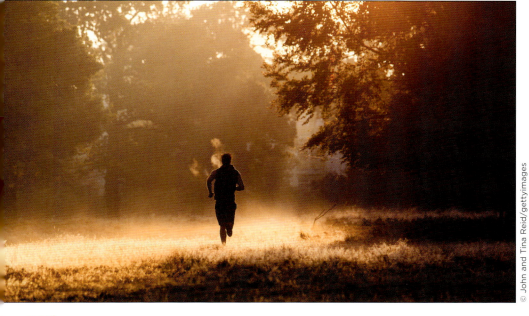

tip: Runners tend to perform best at the time of day they run most often. Be sure to do at least some of your training in the early morning, which is when most races start.

Distance this week: 1   **Weight:**

Distance carried forward: 2.62

25 Monday 85

Where & When:　　　　　　　　　　Distance:
Comments:

26 Tuesday 86

Where & When:　　　　　　　　　　Distance:
Comments:

27 Wednesday 87

Where & When:　　　　　　　　　　Distance:
Comments:

28 Thursday 88

Where & When:　　　　　　　　　　Distance:
Comments:

29 Friday 89

Where & When:　　　　　　　　　　Distance:
Comments:

March

Saturday 30

90

Where & When:　　　　　　　　　　　　　　　Distance:
Comments:

Sunday 31

91

Where & When:　　　　　　　　　　　　　　　Distance:
Comments:

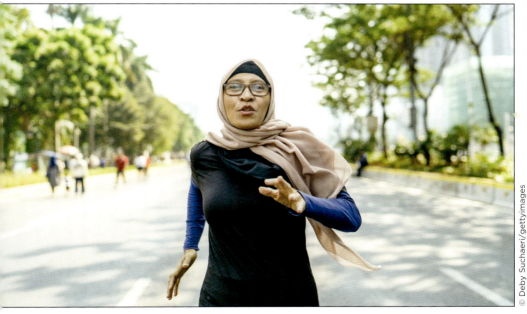

tip: The typical elite runner does eighty percent of their training at low intensity, compared to less than fifty percent for the typical recreational runner. Take a cue from the pros and slow down!

Distance this week:　　　　　　　　　　　　　Weight:

April

SUNDAY	MONDAY	TUESDAY	WEDNESDAY	THURSDAY	FRIDAY	SATURDAY
	1 Easter Monday (Australia, Canada, Ireland, NZ, UK—except Scotland)	2 Last Quarter	3	4	5	6
7	8 New Moon	9 Eid al-Fitr	10	11	12	13
14	15 First Quarter	16	17	18	19	20
21	22 Passover (begins at sundown) Earth Day	23 Full Moon St. George's Day (UK)	24	25 Anzac Day (NZ, Australia)	26	27
28	29	30 Passover ends				

tip: Be sure to use some of your long runs as opportunities to practice your fueling plan for your next race. For maximum performance, drink every ten to fifteen minutes and take in sixty to ninety grams of carbs per hour in the form of energy gels and sports drinks.

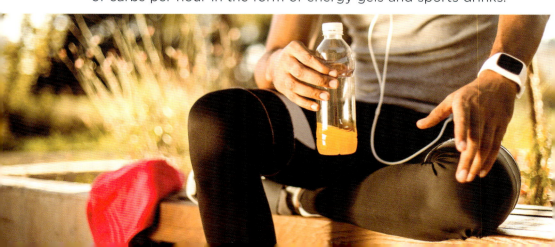

THE PROGRESS TRAP

I started running on April 19, 1983. The date sticks with me because I watched my dad run the Boston Marathon the day before, which made me want to be a runner, too. My first run was a six-miler on the dirt roads surrounding my family's home in rural New Hampshire. I wore a watch and recorded my time.

Two days later I ran the same route again, hoping to better my time, and did. This happened on a Thursday. On Saturday, I went through the same routine, achieving my best time yet. But my next run was a disaster. My legs felt heavy from the first step, and try as I might, I couldn't keep the streak of personal bests going. This was my introduction to the Progress Trap.

Every runner loves progress. To see oneself improve in response to work done on the roads, trails, tracks, and treadmills is deeply satisfying. Progress in running isn't linear, however, and it doesn't happen every day. We know this, yet we are prone to forget. So intoxicating is the thrill of ascent that, despite our better knowledge, we expect continuous improvement, or worse, try to force it.

I coached a runner who liked to train by heart rate. As she got fitter, she found that she was able to go faster at the same low heart rate in easy runs, which made her happy. But the trend couldn't last forever, and when she started experiencing runs in which, perhaps due to fatigue from the heavier training load she was carrying, she actually needed to slow down to stay in the right heart-rate zone, she refused to do so. The result was that she stopped improving and started to slide backward until we had a little talk.

When I see a runner getting sucked into the trap, I deliver good news and bad news. The bad news is that—as they already know (but have temporarily forgotten)—they cannot improve every time they run. The good news is that, even so, every run can contribute to their improvement if they understand and respect its specific purpose. In a well-designed training program, there are different types of runs, each with its own purpose. Even a day off contributes to progress by allowing the body to recover, adapt, and emerge ready for the next challenge.

It's okay to want to improve as much and as quickly as possible. Most runners do. But the secret to maximizing improvement is giving your body what it needs—whether a tough speed workout, a gentle recovery run, or something in between—not testing your body's limits or seeking proof of progress each day. None of us is immune; beware the Progress Trap! ■

Distance carried forward:

1 Monday 92

Where & When: **Distance:**
Comments:

2 Tuesday 93

Where & When: **Distance:**
Comments:

3 Wednesday 94

Where & When: **Distance:**
Comments:

4 Thursday 95

Where & When: **Distance:**
Comments:

5 Friday 96

Where & When: **Distance:**
Comments:

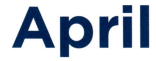

April

97   **Saturday 6**

Where & When: Distance:
Comments:

98   **Sunday 7**

Where & When: Distance:
Comments:

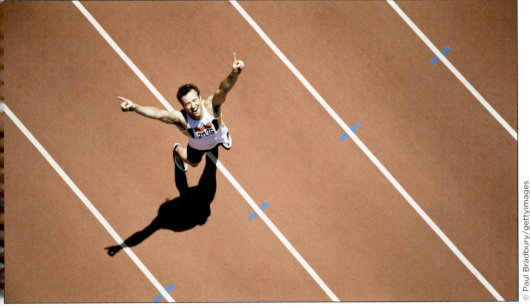

© Paul Bradbury/gettyimages

tip: One of the most powerful things you can do to stay motivated for running is to monitor your progress. Seeing quantitative proof that you're improving will fire you up to keep improving.

Distance this week: Weight:

Distance carried forward:

8 Monday 99

Where & When: **Distance:**
Comments:

9 Tuesday 100

Where & When: **Distance:**
Comments:

10 Wednesday 101

Where & When: **Distance:**
Comments:

11 Thursday 102

Where & When: **Distance:**
Comments:

12 Friday 103

Where & When: **Distance:**
Comments:

April

104

Saturday 13

Where & When: Distance:
Comments:

105

Sunday 14

Where & When: Distance:
Comments:

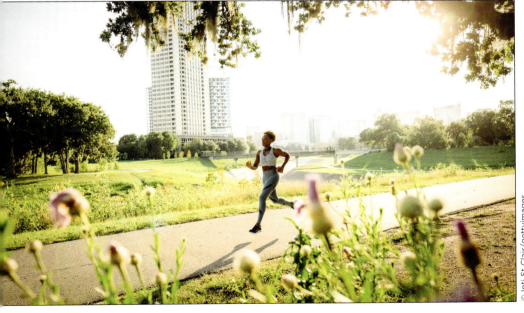

tip: It may not be the buzziest word, but "consistency" truly is the most important factor in run training. Success comes not from surviving a few heroic workouts but from stringing together a whole bunch of good runs.

Distance this week: Weight:

Distance carried forward:

15 Monday 106

Where & When: **Distance:**
Comments:

16 Tuesday 107

Where & When: **Distance:**
Comments:

17 Wednesday 108

Where & When: **Distance:**
Comments:

18 Thursday 109

Where & When: **Distance:**
Comments:

19 Friday 110

Where & When: **Distance:**
Comments:

April

11

Saturday 20

Where & When:　　　　　　　　　　　　　　Distance:
Comments:

12

Sunday 21

Where & When:　　　　　　　　　　　　　　Distance:
Comments:

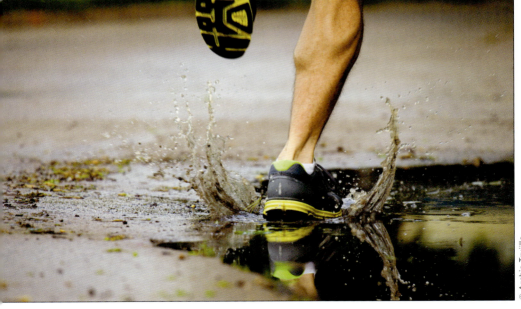

tip: April showers bring puddles. Before you lace up for a run that's likely to be wet, slather some petroleum jelly on your feet to prevent chafing.

Distance this week:　　　　　　　　　　　　Weight:

Distance carried forward:

22 Monday 113

Where & When: **Distance:**
Comments:

23 Tuesday 114

Where & When: **Distance:**
Comments:

24 Wednesday 115

Where & When: **Distance:**
Comments:

25 Thursday 116

Where & When: **Distance:**
Comments:

26 Friday 117

Where & When: **Distance:**
Comments:

April

Saturday 27
18 (5k)

Where & When: Distance:
Comments:

Sunday 28
19

Where & When: Distance:
Comments:

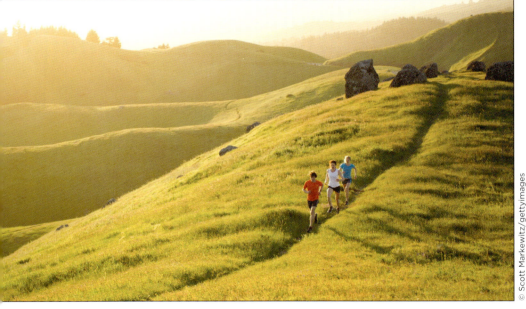
© Scott Markewitz/gettyimages

tip: Try to train on trails at least once a week. Not only is it fun, but the varied terrain will test your balance, agility, and stability in ways that road running doesn't, making your running fitness more well-rounded.

Distance this week: Weight:

Distance carried forward: _____

29 Monday   120

_____
_____

Where & When: _____ Distance: _____
Comments: _____

30 Tuesday   12?

_____
_____

Where & When: _____ Distance: _____
Comments: _____

1 Wednesday   122

_____
_____

Where & When: _____ Distance: _____
Comments: _____

2 Thursday   123

_____
_____

Where & When: _____ Distance: _____
Comments: _____

3 Friday   124

_____
_____

Where & When: _____ Distance: _____
Comments: _____

Apr/May

25 **Saturday 4**

Where & When: Distance:
Comments:

26 **Sunday 5**

Where & When: Distance:
Comments:

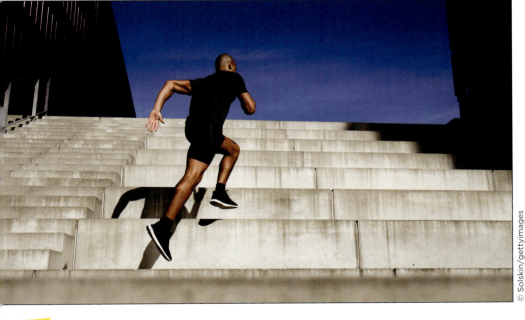

© Solskin/gettyimages

tip: Running increases the body's needs for a number of essential micronutrients, including riboflavin and vitamin B6. A high-quality diet based on fruits and vegetables will meet these elevated requirements.

Distance this week: Weight:

May

SUNDAY	MONDAY	TUESDAY	WEDNESDAY	THURSDAY	FRIDAY	SATURDAY
			1	2	3 Holy Friday (Orthodox)	4
			☾ Last Quarter			
5 Easter (Orthodox) Yom HaShoah (begins at sundown)	6 May Day (Australia—NT) Labour Day (Australia—QLD) Early May Bank Holiday (Ireland, UK)	7	8 ● New Moon	9	10	11
12 Mother's Day (USA, Australia, Canada, NZ)	13	14	15 ☽ First Quarter	16	17	18 Armed Forces Day (USA)
19	20	21	22	23 ○ Full Moon	24	25
	Victoria Day (Canada)					
26	27 Memorial Day (USA) Bank Holiday (UK)	28	29	30 ☾ Last Quarter	31	

tip: Most running injuries are preceded by abrupt increases in training load. To stay healthy, limit yourself to gradual upticks in mileage and intensity.

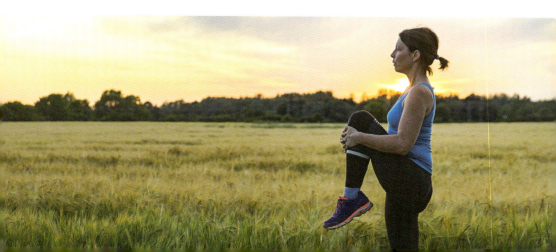

NO FINISH LINE

Every runner has goals. Few of us, however, spend much time reflecting on those goals. We set them, pursue them, celebrate their achievement (or lament their nonachievement), and move on. There's nothing wrong with any of this, but have you ever stopped to wonder what's the point of it all?

My first big running goal was to break five minutes in the mile. As a high school freshman, I was fixated on joining the sub-five club, but when I broke through that magical barrier toward the end of the outdoor track season, I forgot all about it and immediately set my sights on going under 4:50. Soon 4:40 became the new magic number.

With few exceptions, all running goals are like this. In themselves, the numbers mean nothing. If they did, every sub-five-minute mile I ran would have been as satisfying as the one before, even when I reached the point of running two in a row without stopping. The goals we set as runners are meaningful only as symbols of our improvement. The moment we achieve them, they lose significance, and we must choose new goals.

When you look at it from this perspective, there is only one goal, and that is improvement. But what happens when we inevitably stop improving? Trick question! We never stop, at least not if we understand what *improvement* really means.

As I see it, there are two ways to improve in running. One is to get faster; the other, to gain mastery. No runner gets faster forever, but mastery is nothing more than the ability to make good decisions—when to push and when to rest, when to speed up and when to slow down, when to give yourself a pep talk and when a scolding—and this ability grows through experience and learning, which have no limit.

Some dislike the word "mastery," which carries connotations of domination and ownership. I get that, but I also can't think of a better word for the sense of assured control that comes with experience and learning in running. Speaking for myself, I really did feel as though I "owned" my running more and more as the years and the miles piled up. I would stand at the start line and know I would run a smart race, or I would pull up lame in a workout and know I would be okay in a few days, having done it before. It's a good feeling.

Religious scholar James Carse coined the terms "finite games" and "infinite games" in reference to these two ways of improving. "A finite game is played for the purpose of winning," he wrote, "an infinite game for the purpose of continuing the play." I encourage all runners to approach the sport as an infinite game, one with no finish line. ■

Distance carried forward:

6 Monday 127

Where & When: Distance:
Comments:

7 Tuesday 128

Where & When: Distance:
Comments:

8 Wednesday 129

Where & When: Distance:
Comments:

9 Thursday 130

Where & When: Distance:
Comments:

10 Friday 131

Where & When: Distance:
Comments:

May

Saturday 11
132

Where & When: Distance:
Comments:

Sunday 12
133

Where & When: Distance:
Comments:

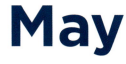

tip: It takes time to reacclimate to running in warm weather. Don't get carried away on the first summerlike day of spring!

Distance this week: Weight:

Distance carried forward: _____

13 Monday   134

_____
_____

Where & When: _____ **Distance:** _____
Comments: _____

14 Tuesday   135

_____
_____

Where & When: _____ **Distance:** _____
Comments: _____

15 Wednesday   136

_____
_____

Where & When: _____ **Distance:** _____
Comments: _____

16 Thursday   137

_____
_____

Where & When: _____ **Distance:** _____
Comments: _____

17 Friday   138

_____
_____

Where & When: _____ **Distance:** _____
Comments: _____

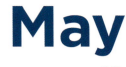

May

Saturday 18

139

Where & When: Distance:
Comments:

Sunday 19

140

Where & When: Distance:
Comments:

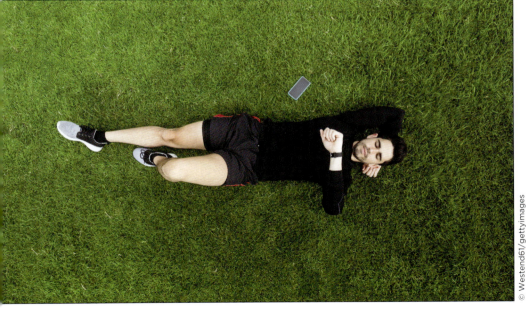

tip: Recovery is about the fundamentals: healthy diet, quality sleep, relaxation, and stress management. Compression boots, cryotherapy, and other expensive recovery tools won't help you if you aren't taking care of the basics.

Distance this week: Weight:

Distance carried forward: _____

20 Monday 141

Where & When: _____ Distance: _____
Comments: _____

21 Tuesday 142

Where & When: _____ Distance: _____
Comments: _____

22 Wednesday 143

Where & When: _____ Distance: _____
Comments: _____

23 Thursday 144

Where & When: _____ Distance: _____
Comments: _____

24 Friday 145

Where & When: _____ Distance: _____
Comments: _____

May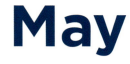

146   **Saturday 25**

Where & When: Distance:
Comments:

147   **Sunday 26**

Where & When: Distance:
Comments:

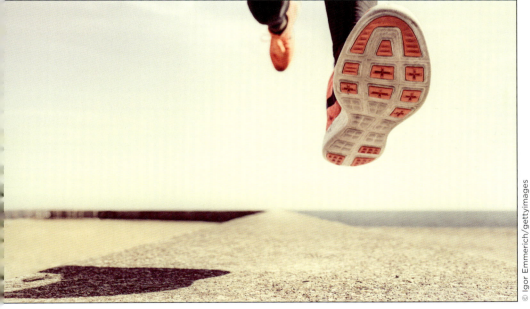

tip: Be sure to track the mileage you put on your running shoes and replace them at the manufacturer's recommended frequency. This will help reduce injury risk.

Distance this week: Weight:

Distance carried forward:

27 Monday 148

Where & When: **Distance:**
Comments:

28 Tuesday 149

Where & When: **Distance:**
Comments:

29 Wednesday 150

Where & When: **Distance:**
Comments:

30 Thursday 151

Where & When: **Distance:**
Comments:

31 Friday 152

Where & When: **Distance:**
Comments:

May/Jun

153   **Saturday 1**

Where & When: Distance:
Comments:

154   **Sunday 2**

Where & When: Distance:
Comments:

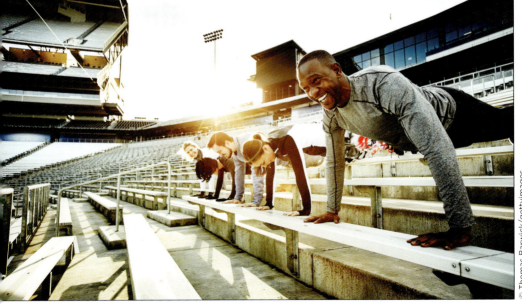

© Thomas Barwick/gettyimages

tip: Make your training as enjoyable as possible in choosing routes, workouts, training partners, music, and gear. The more you enjoy your training, the more you'll get out of it.

Distance this week: Weight:

June

SUNDAY	MONDAY	TUESDAY	WEDNESDAY	THURSDAY	FRIDAY	SATURDAY
						1
2	3 King's Birthday (NZ) Bank Holiday (Ireland)	4	5	6 ● New Moon	7	8
9	10 King's Birthday (Australia—except QLD, WA)	11	12	13	14 ◐ First Quarter Flag Day (USA)	15
16 Eid al-Adha Father's Day (USA, Canada, Ireland, UK)	17	18	19 Juneteenth (USA)	20 Summer Solstice	21 National Indigenous Peoples Day (Canada)	22 ○ Full Moon
23	24	25	26	27	28 ◑ Last Quarter	29
30						

tip: Running is more of a participatory sport than a spectator sport, but being a fan of professional running can inspire your own training and racing. Treat yourself to the occasional elite competition and see if cheering on the best in the world doesn't fire you up.

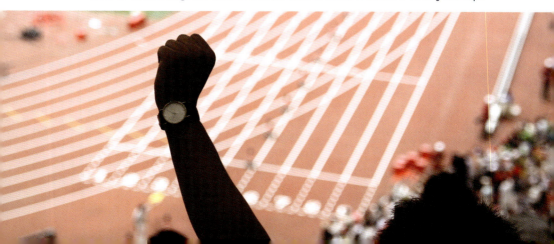

WHAT'S YOUR STORY?

When I was nine years old (two years shy of my first run), I told my parents I wanted to be an author one day, and I've been writing ever since. Perhaps this is why I've always looked at my running journey as a story. All stories have themes, and the overarching theme I've applied to my athletic narrative is redemption.

In high school I became what is often called a head case, so fearful of the pain of racing that I did shameful things to avoid it (faking injuries, coasting through races). The problem became so severe that it ultimately caused me to quit the sport forever—or so I thought. Fate had other plans, and when I returned to running in my late twenties, I was motivated by a powerful desire to redeem myself—to write a new ending to the story, in which I played the hero instead of the goat. I'm happy to report that I succeeded in this quest, scripting a second act of my life as a runner that has been infinitely more satisfying than the first.

I'm not alone in looking at my athletic pursuits through a narrative lens. Psychologists have learned that most athletes storify their sports careers to some extent, and that, in particular, elite athletes do so in ways that contribute to their success. British researchers found that elite track and field athletes made sense of their experiences with injury through one of several self-chosen themes. More recently, German scientists have shown that high-achieving athletes, scientists, and musicians narrativized their careers through similar themes, which they named Searching for the Spotlight, Straightforward Career, Overcoming Obstacles, Riding the Waves, and Applying Effort.

French sociologist Pierre Bourdieu coined the term *illusio* to refer to the uniquely human practice of finding meaning in our lives through story. An important thing to understand about illusio is that it's a skill, and like any skill, it can be improved through intentional practice. A study published in *Frontiers in Psychology* reported that elite athletes were marked by a "low past negative time perspective" and an overall "future time perspective," whereas non-elite athletes had the opposite traits. This suggests that athletic success is aided by telling stories focused on creating a positive future rather than dwelling on a negative past. Though far from elite, I like to think this is what I've been doing in chasing redemption as a runner. How about you? What's your story? ∎

Distance carried forward:

3 Monday 155

Where & When: Distance:
Comments:

4 Tuesday 156

Where & When: Distance:
Comments:

5 Wednesday 157

Where & When: Distance:
Comments:

6 Thursday 158

Where & When: Distance:
Comments:

7 Friday 159

Where & When: Distance:
Comments:

June

160

Saturday 8

Where & When: **Distance:**
Comments:

161

Sunday 9

Where & When: **Distance:**
Comments:

© Jordan Siemans/gettyimages

tip: Starting a daily run streak can be an effective way to break out of a motivational rut. And what better time to start one than National Running Day (June 5th)?

Distance this week: **Weight:**

Distance carried forward: _____

10 Monday   162

_____
_____

Where & When: _____ Distance: _____
Comments: _____

11 Tuesday   163

_____
_____

Where & When: _____ Distance: _____
Comments: _____

12 Wednesday   164

_____
_____

Where & When: _____ Distance: _____
Comments: _____

13 Thursday   165

_____
_____

Where & When: _____ Distance: _____
Comments: _____

14 Friday   166

_____
_____

Where & When: _____ Distance: _____
Comments: _____

June

167

Saturday 15

Where & When: Distance:
Comments:

168

Sunday 16

Where & When: Distance:
Comments:

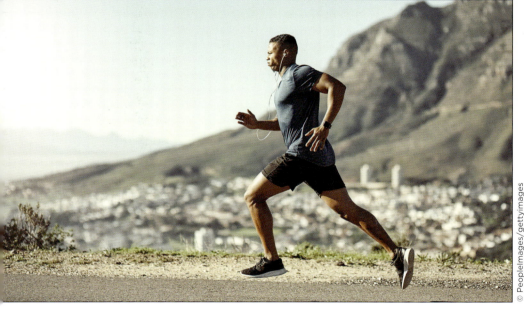

tip: The true measure of running fitness is the ability to run fast with tired legs. You can improve this ability with progression runs, where you start at an easy pace and speed up incrementally.

Distance this week: Weight:

Distance carried forward: _____

17 Monday   169

_____
_____
_____

Where & When: _____ **Distance:** _____
Comments: _____

18 Tuesday   170

_____
_____
_____

Where & When: _____ **Distance:** _____
Comments: _____

19 Wednesday   171

_____
_____
_____

Where & When: _____ **Distance:** _____
Comments: _____

20 Thursday   172

_____
_____
_____

Where & When: _____ **Distance:** _____
Comments: _____

21 Friday   173

_____
_____
_____

Where & When: _____ **Distance:** _____
Comments: _____

June

Saturday 22

174

Where & When: Distance:
Comments:

Sunday 23

175

Where & When: Distance:
Comments:

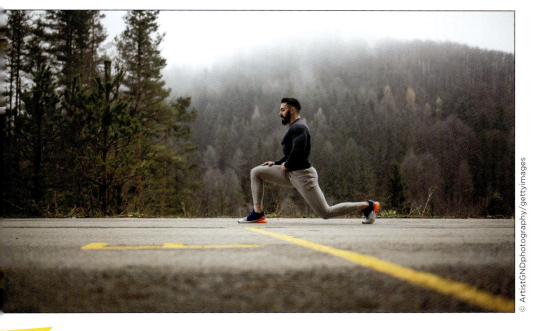

tip: The ideal pre-race warm-up has four parts: Start with a few dynamic stretches such as walking lunges, then do a little jogging followed by a handful of technique drills, then finish up with a couple of short, relaxed sprints. Now you're ready to race!

Distance this week: Weight:

Distance carried forward: _____

24 Monday 176

_____
_____

Where & When: _____ Distance: _____
Comments: _____

25 Tuesday 177

_____
_____

Where & When: _____ Distance: _____
Comments: _____

26 Wednesday 178

_____
_____

Where & When: _____ Distance: _____
Comments: _____

27 Thursday 179

_____
_____

Where & When: _____ Distance: _____
Comments: _____

28 Friday 180

_____
_____

Where & When: _____ Distance: _____
Comments: _____

June

Saturday 29

181

Where & When: **Distance:**
Comments:

Sunday 30

182

Where & When: **Distance:**
Comments:

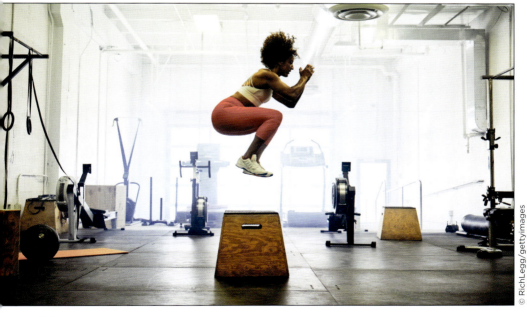

tip: Every runner feels the same amount of discomfort when pushing hard. What distinguishes mentally tough runners is how they interpret the discomfort they're feeling.

Distance this week: **Weight:**

July

SUNDAY	MONDAY	TUESDAY	WEDNESDAY	THURSDAY	FRIDAY	SATURDAY
	1 Canada Day	2	3	4 Independence Day (USA)	5 ● New Moon	6
7	8	9	10	11	12	13 ◐ First Quarter
14	15	16	17	18	19	20
21	22	23	24	25	26	27
28 ○ Full Moon	29	30	31			
◑ Last Quarter						

tip: If you eat something within forty-five minutes of completing each workout, you will recover quicker and perform better in your next run. Include carbohydrates to replenish fuel stores, protein to repair damaged muscle tissue, and fluid to rehydrate.

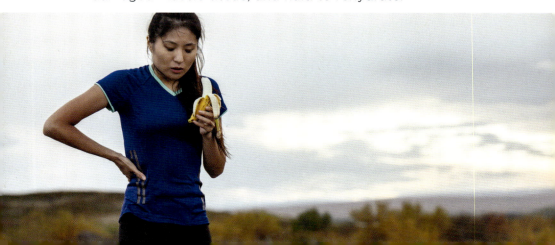

NO COMPARISON

Like all sports, running invites comparisons. The measurements that define the sport—distance, time, pace—have no meaning except inasmuch as we use them to make comparisons. Achievements such as completing your longest run ever and qualifying for the Boston Marathon feel good because they compare favorably to other things.

Comparisons can be dangerous, though. Theodore Roosevelt famously called them "the thief of joy." I've known too many runners who get woefully down on themselves after trying and failing to BQ, for example. When runners measure themselves against other runners, they don't always measure up, and there goes their joy.

Is the solution, then, to measure only against oneself? You might think so, but these comparisons can also be fraught. Some runners I've coached have become demoralized when their training was disrupted by injury or some other factor and their numbers dropped, falling short of their previous standards.

The true solution to the dangers associated with comparisons is to stop making comparisons. *Just kidding!* That's no solution either. The smart way to keep comparisons from stealing your joy is by exercising what psychologists call logical attribution, and what the rest of us call keeping things in perspective. If you think about it, comparisons only steal our joy when we lose perspective, illogically attributing the cause of not measuring up to things beyond our control.

Not every runner can qualify for the Boston Marathon. Those who don't have no logical reason to get down on themselves for missing the mark. As a coach, I never dissuade a runner from going after a big goal just because I doubt their ability to achieve it. With the right perspective, the experience of reaching for a high mark is extremely rewarding regardless of whether the mark is reached. Failure sucks but not as much as never trying.

Some runners lose their joy when age begins to slow them down. Illogical! Talk about things beyond your control—that's why races have age divisions, and why age-graded performance calculators can be found online. Even when you can't do quite as well as you used to, you can do well—perhaps better than ever—all things considered. It's a matter of perspective. ■

Distance carried forward:

1 Monday 183

Where & When: **Distance:**
Comments:

2 Tuesday 184

Where & When: **Distance:**
Comments:

3 Wednesday 185

Where & When: **Distance:**
Comments:

4 Thursday 186

Where & When: **Distance:**
Comments:

5 Friday 187

Where & When: **Distance:**
Comments:

July

188 **Saturday 6**

Where & When: Distance:
Comments:

189 **Sunday 7**

Where & When: Distance:
Comments:

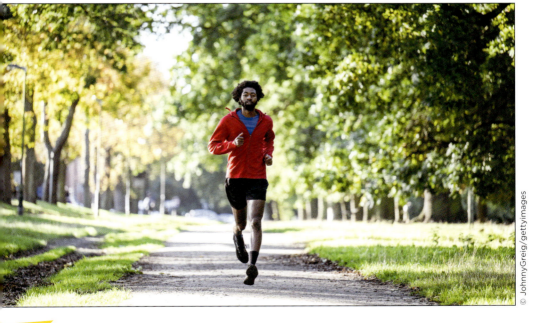

tip: The importance of long runs in marathon training is somewhat exaggerated. Studies suggest that average weekly mileage has a bigger impact on marathon performance than the distance of the longest single run.

Distance this week: Weight:

Distance carried forward:

8 Monday 190

Where & When: **Distance:**
Comments:

9 Tuesday 191

Where & When: **Distance:**
Comments:

10 Wednesday 192

Where & When: **Distance:**
Comments:

11 Thursday 193

Where & When: **Distance:**
Comments:

12 Friday 194

Where & When: **Distance:**
Comments:

July

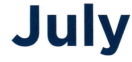

Saturday 13

195

Where & When: Distance:
Comments:

Sunday 14

196

Where & When: Distance:
Comments:

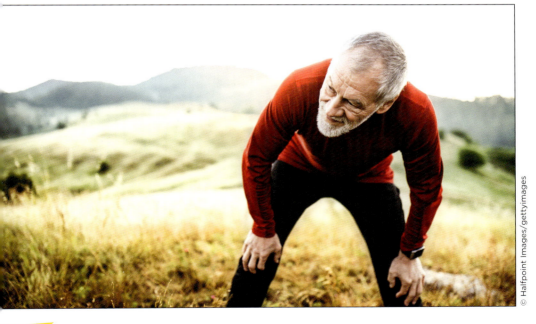

tip: When you feel an injury coming on, practice "incremental retreat," altering your training as little as necessary to allow the issue to resolve. Take a break from speed work, for example, or switch to softer surfaces.

Distance this week: Weight:

Distance carried forward:

15 Monday 197

Where & When: **Distance:**
Comments:

16 Tuesday 198

Where & When: **Distance:**
Comments:

17 Wednesday 199

Where & When: **Distance:**
Comments:

18 Thursday 200

Where & When: **Distance:**
Comments:

19 Friday 201

Where & When: **Distance:**
Comments:

July

202

Saturday 20

Where & When: Distance:
Comments:

203

Sunday 21

Where & When: Distance:
Comments:

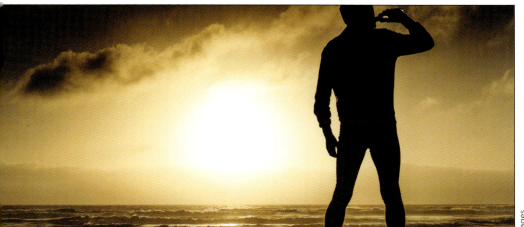

tip: Drink according to your thirst during longer workouts and races. Forcing yourself to drink more than your body asks for can result in discomfort. Research has shown that *ad libitum* drinking optimizes both performance and thermoregulation.

Distance this week: Weight:

Distance carried forward: _____

22 Monday   204

_____
_____

Where & When: _____ **Distance:** _____
Comments: _____

23 Tuesday   205

_____
_____

Where & When: _____ **Distance:** _____
Comments: _____

24 Wednesday   206

_____
_____

Where & When: _____ **Distance:** _____
Comments: _____

25 Thursday   207

_____
_____

Where & When: _____ **Distance:** _____
Comments: _____

26 Friday   208

_____
_____

Where & When: _____ **Distance:** _____
Comments: _____

July

Saturday 27

209

Where & When: Distance:
Comments:

Sunday 28

210

Where & When: Distance:
Comments:

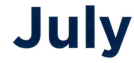

tip: Running in the heat is proven to increase performance by boosting blood volume. Just don't overdo it!

Distance this week: Weight:

© Pete Saloutos/gettyimages

Distance carried forward: _____

29 Monday 211

_____
_____

Where & When: _____ **Distance:** _____
Comments: _____

30 Tuesday 212

_____
_____

Where & When: _____ **Distance:** _____
Comments: _____

31 Wednesday 213

_____
_____

Where & When: _____ **Distance:** _____
Comments: _____

1 Thursday 214

_____
_____

Where & When: _____ **Distance:** _____
Comments: _____

2 Friday 215

_____
_____

Where & When: _____ **Distance:** _____
Comments: _____

Jul/Aug

Saturday 3

216

Where & When: Distance:
Comments:

Sunday 4

217

Where & When: Distance:
Comments:

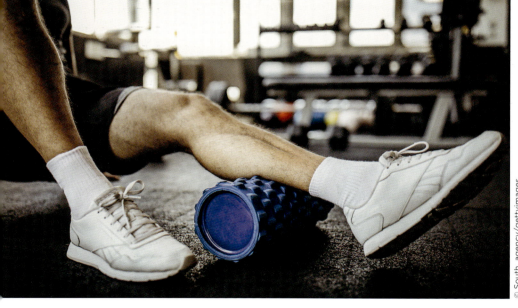

© South_agency/gettyimages

tip: Foam rolling can aid your running by releasing tight spots in your muscles. Just a few minutes of rolling out your legs after each run will make a noticeable difference in how you feel and move.

Distance this week: Weight:

August

SUNDAY	MONDAY	TUESDAY	WEDNESDAY	THURSDAY	FRIDAY	SATURDAY
				1	2	3
4 ● New Moon	5 Bank Holiday (Ireland, UK—Scotland, Australia—NSW) Picnic Day (Australia—NT)	6	7	8	9	10
11	12 ◐ First Quarter	13	14	15	16	17
18	19 ○ Full Moon	20	21	22	23	24
25	26 ◑ Last Quarter Bank Holiday (UK—except Scotland)	27	28	29	30	31

tip: Mindfulness meditation is a powerful tool for runners that is proven to improve perceived effort tolerance and mental focus. It also reduces stress and improves overall subjective well-being. Why wait? Meditate!

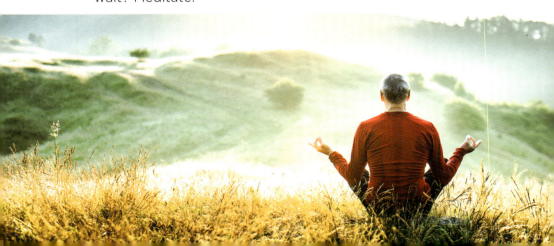

THE WORSE, THE BETTER

The longest marathon I ever ran was the Rockin' K Trail Marathon in Kansas.

I know what you're thinking: All marathons are the same distance! What's this guy talking about? That's true—but only if I don't get lost.

I knew I was in for a long day well before I came upon the remote Gate 6 aid station from the wrong direction, having missed a turn two miles back. The start of the race was delayed by a lightning storm. At five miles, I was nearly swept downstream when I lost my footing at a river crossing but was saved by the outstretched arm of a fellow runner. I slipped again at the top of a steep and muddy embankment and sledded the whole way down on my rear end. By the time I reached the mirage-like aid station, where I was informed by the race director that I would have to turn back and repeat the loop in the proper direction, I looked like a man who'd been dragged behind a horse.

Weirdly, though, I was having a *blast*. I found myself looking forward to, even hoping for, the next mishap, of which there were plenty, including a bothersome pebble in my shoe that turned out to be in my sock. I couldn't wait to tell my wife the story of my thirty-mile marathon when (or if) I made it back to our hotel.

We all want things to go well when we start a race or other important run. That's only human. But they don't always go well, and sometimes a whole bunch of things go really wrong, as they did for me at the Rockin' K Trail Marathon. The mistake we sometimes make is allowing ourselves to become emotionally dependent on things going well, which ruins the experience if they don't. I didn't make this mistake in Kansas, and that made all the difference.

With the right attitude, every run can be a good experience. When things go well, we get to enjoy a flow state and peak performance. And when they don't go well, we get to broaden our definition of success, as I did in my longest marathon. I think this is what Tom Warren was getting at when he told *Sports Illustrated* writer Barry McDermott (before winning the second-ever Ironman triathlon in 1979), "I'm only in mediocre shape right now, but sometimes it's better that way." Tom knew going into the competition that, win or lose, he was in for a challenging adventure, and he embraced it. ■

Distance carried forward:

5 Monday 218

Where & When: **Distance:**
Comments:

6 Tuesday 219

Where & When: **Distance:**
Comments:

7 Wednesday 220

Where & When: **Distance:**
Comments:

8 Thursday 221

Where & When: **Distance:**
Comments:

9 Friday 222

Where & When: **Distance:**
Comments:

August

223 **Saturday 10**

Where & When: Distance:
Comments:

224 **Sunday 11**

Where & When: Distance:
Comments:

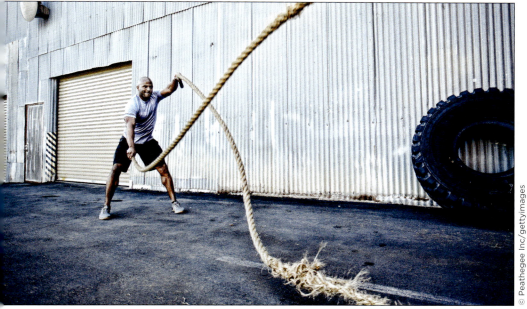

tip: People enjoy exercising more when they mix things up, doing different types of workouts in other environments instead of repeating the same thing day after day. Next time you find your running getting stale, add some variety!

Distance this week: Weight:

Distance carried forward:

12 Monday 225

Where & When: Distance:
Comments:

13 Tuesday 226

Where & When: Distance:
Comments:

14 Wednesday 227

Where & When: Distance:
Comments:

15 Thursday 228

Where & When: Distance:
Comments:

16 Friday 229

Where & When: Distance:
Comments:

August

Saturday 17

230

Where & When: Distance:
Comments:

Sunday 18

231

Where & When: Distance:
Comments:

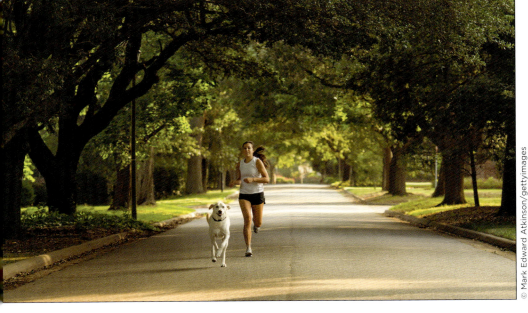

tip: The term "recovery run" is a bit of a misnomer. The purpose of these short, low-intensity runs is not to accelerate recovery from previous training but to offer a gentle training stimulus that doesn't interfere with your recovery from prior training.

Distance this week: Weight:

Distance carried forward: _____

19 Monday   232

_____
_____

Where & When: _____ **Distance:** _____
Comments: _____

20 Tuesday   233

_____
_____

Where & When: _____ **Distance:** _____
Comments: _____

21 Wednesday   234

_____
_____

Where & When: _____ **Distance:** _____
Comments: _____

22 Thursday   235

_____
_____

Where & When: _____ **Distance:** _____
Comments: _____

23 Friday   236

_____
_____

Where & When: _____ **Distance:** _____
Comments: _____

August

Saturday 24

237

Where & When: Distance:
Comments:

Sunday 25

238

Where & When: Distance:
Comments:

tip: Never try to do consciously something you can do automatically when running! Runners become less efficient when they merely think about their breathing, even when they're not trying to control or change it.

Distance this week: Weight:

© Erik Isakson/gettyimages

Distance carried forward:

26 Monday 239

Where & When: **Distance:**
Comments:

27 Tuesday 240

Where & When: **Distance:**
Comments:

28 Wednesday 241

Where & When: **Distance:**
Comments:

29 Thursday 242

Where & When: **Distance:**
Comments:

30 Friday 243

Where & When: **Distance:**
Comments:

Aug/Sep

Saturday 31

244

Where & When: Distance:
Comments:

Sunday 1

245

Where & When: Distance:
Comments:

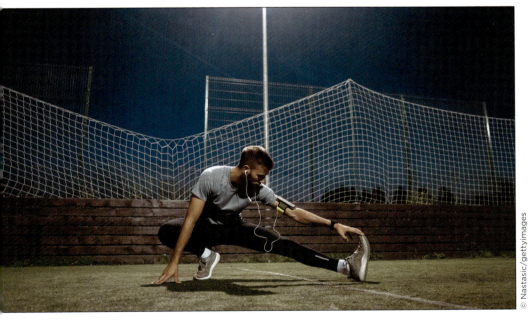

tip: If you spend a lot of timing sitting during the day, be sure to do one or more dynamic stretches, such as side lunges, before you head out the door. These will make the transition from rest to running a little gentler on your body.

Distance this week: Weight:

September

SUNDAY	MONDAY	TUESDAY	WEDNESDAY	THURSDAY	FRIDAY	SATURDAY
1 Father's Day (Australia, NZ)	2 Labor Day (USA, Canada)	3 ● New Moon	4	5	6	7
8	9	10	11 ◐ First Quarter	12	13	14
15	16	17	18 ○ Full Moon	19	20	21 U.N. International Day of Peace
22	23	24 ◑ Last Quarter	25	26	27	28
29 Autumnal Equinox	30 King's Birthday (Australia—WA)					

tip: Try to do at least some of your runs on terrain similar to the event you're preparing for, whether flat roads, hilly trails, or a rubberized track. The body does best on what it is most accustomed to!

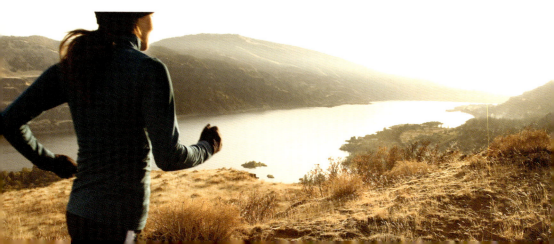

IT'S NEVER ALL BAD

A lot can go wrong in an Ironman triathlon. In my first, it happened early, when a vicious cramp in my right calf brought me to a sudden stop less than one hundred yards into a 2.4-mile open-water swim in Wisconsin's Lake Monona. Later, when I mounted my bike to begin the one hundred and twelve-mile second leg of the event, I made the unhappy discovery that the cramp had in fact injured the affected muscle, my pain intensifying with each turn of the cranks.

By the time I started the running portion—a full marathon—the discomfort had spread across the entire back side of my leg. As I hobbled on, my foot went dead, a pins-and-needles sort of numbness creeping slowly up my shank and into my thigh. Unable to feel the impact between my right foot and the pavement, I was forced to keep my eyes rooted on the road beneath me to maintain my balance.

It was then I experienced a revelation that has stayed with me ever since. Desperate to take my mind off the crisis in my leg, I swiveled my attention outward. A beautiful September afternoon surrounded me, and despite my distress, I found I was able to appreciate its pleasant warmth. Refocusing inward, I realized that, apart from a frozen leg, I felt pretty good for a man who'd been exercising at high intensity for the past nine hours. All in all, I had very little to complain about. Here I was, in the best shape of my life, doing something I loved, on track to achieve a goal I'd worked hard for, flanked by athletic comrades, cheered on by our families and friends and the good people of Madison. "It's never all bad," I told myself as I finished the race with a dopey grin on my face.

This was more than twenty years ago. In all the time since then, I haven't changed my mind about this simple truth. I call upon it whenever pain or misfortune threatens to spoil an experience, athletic or not, and it always works. Even when something very bad is happening, or more than one bad thing, there's always space in our minds and hearts to enjoy and be grateful for the good things also happening. ■

Distance carried forward:

2 Monday 246

Where & When: **Distance:**
Comments:

3 Tuesday 247

Where & When: **Distance:**
Comments:

4 Wednesday 248

Where & When: **Distance:**
Comments:

5 Thursday 249

Where & When: **Distance:**
Comments:

6 Friday 250

Where & When: **Distance:**
Comments:

September

Saturday 7

251

Where & When: Distance:
Comments:

Sunday 8

252

Where & When: Distance:
Comments:

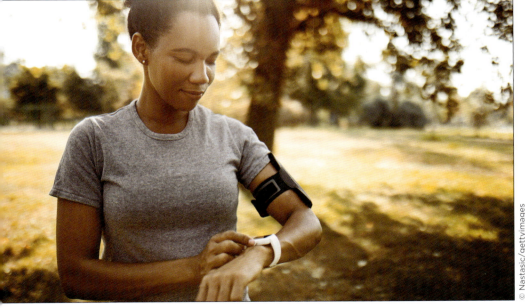

tip: Technology should be a tool, never a crutch, in your training. Successful runners are really good at listening to their bodies. Overreliance on devices can impede development of this important ability.

Distance this week: Weight:

Distance carried forward:

9 Monday 253

Where & When: **Distance:**
Comments:

10 Tuesday 254

Where & When: **Distance:**
Comments:

11 Wednesday 255

Where & When: **Distance:**
Comments:

12 Thursday 256

Where & When: **Distance:**
Comments:

13 Friday 257

Where & When: **Distance:**
Comments:

September

258   **Saturday 14**

Where & When: Distance:
Comments:

259   **Sunday 15**

Where & When: Distance:
Comments:

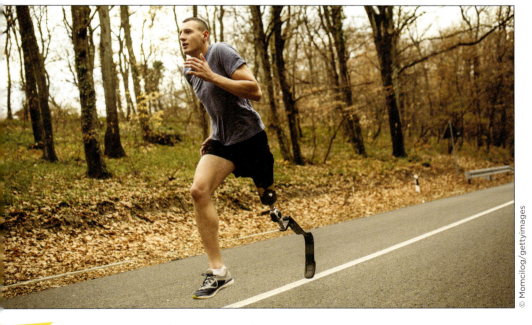

© Momcilog/gettyimages

tip: Maintaining a steady pace yields the best results in races. Use your training to determine the fastest pace you think you can sustain for the full distance of your next race and then stick to it (allowing for some variation on hills, of course).

Distance this week: Weight:

Distance carried forward: _____

16 Monday   260

_____
_____

Where & When: _____ Distance: _____
Comments: _____

17 Tuesday   261

_____
_____

Where & When: _____ Distance: _____
Comments: _____

18 Wednesday   262

_____
_____

Where & When: _____ Distance: _____
Comments: _____

19 Thursday   263

_____
_____

Where & When: _____ Distance: _____
Comments: _____

20 Friday   264

_____
_____

Where & When: _____ Distance: _____
Comments: _____

September

265   **Saturday 21**

Where & When: Distance:
Comments:

266   **Sunday 22**

Where & When: Distance:
Comments:

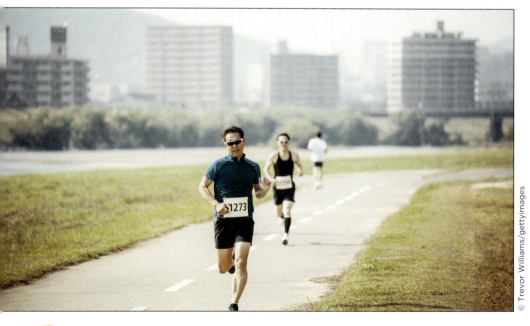

tip: Iron deficiency is common among runners, so be sure to have a doctor check your levels regularly. If you feel lethargic in your training, try eating more iron-rich foods, such as shellfish, leafy greens, legumes, dried fruit, and teff, or take an iron supplement.

Distance this week: Weight:

Distance carried forward:

23 Monday   267

Where & When: **Distance:**
Comments:

24 Tuesday   268

Where & When: **Distance:**
Comments:

25 Wednesday   269

Where & When: **Distance:**
Comments:

26 Thursday   270

Where & When: **Distance:**
Comments:

27 Friday   271

Where & When: **Distance**
Comments:

September

272   **Saturday 28**

Where & When: Distance:
Comments:

273   **Sunday 29**

Where & When: Distance:
Comments:

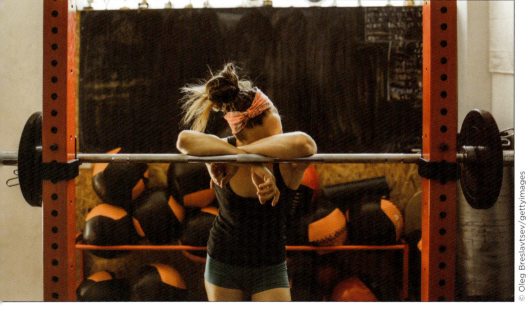

© Oleg Breslavtsev/gettyimages

tip: Don't let a single bad workout negatively impact your confidence. It's our best workouts that tell us how fit we truly are, not our worst ones.

Distance this week: Weight:

Distance carried forward: _____

30 Monday 274

_____
_____

Where & When: _____ Distance: _____
Comments: _____

1 Tuesday 275

_____
_____

Where & When: _____ Distance: _____
Comments: _____

2 Wednesday 276

_____
_____

Where & When: _____ Distance: _____
Comments: _____

3 Thursday 277

_____
_____

Where & When: _____ Distance: _____
Comments: _____

4 Friday 278

_____
_____

Where & When: _____ Distance: _____
Comments: _____

Sep/Oct

279   **Saturday 5**

Where & When: **Distance:**
Comments:

280   **Sunday 6**

Where & When: **Distance:**
Comments:

© Grant Faint/gettyimages

tip: Next time you find yourself unmotivated to run, try the "ten-minute trick." Commit to running for just ten minutes. This will at least get you out the door, and after ten minutes of running you'll probably decide you want to keep going.

Distance this week: **Weight:**

October

SUNDAY	MONDAY	TUESDAY	WEDNESDAY	THURSDAY	FRIDAY	SATURDAY
		1	2 ● New Moon, Rosh Hashanah (begins at sundown)	3	4 Rosh Hashanah ends	5
6	7 Labour Day (Australia—ACT, SA, NSW) King's Birthday (Australia—QLD)	8	9	10 ◐ First Quarter	11 Yom Kippur (begins at sundown)	12
13	14 Columbus Day (USA) Indigenous Peoples' Day (USA) Thanksgiving (Canada)	15	16	17 ○ Full Moon	18	19
20	21	22	23	24 ◑ Last Quarter United Nations Day	25	26
27	28 Labour Day (NZ) Bank Holiday (Ireland)	29	30	31 Diwali Halloween		

tip: Elite runners practice "chunking," mentally dividing races and workouts into smaller steps and focusing on completing one step at a time. When you're miles from the finish line, think of the next water station as your goal.

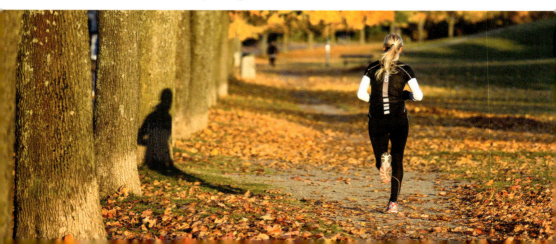

ASKING FOR A FRIEND

Raise your hand if you've ever made a dumb decision that hurt your running! Okay, we can all put our hands down.

Like you, I've made my share of boneheaded mistakes over the years, even though I'm supposed to be some kind of expert. For example, I once decided it was a good idea to race the Orange County Marathon two weeks after a disappointing outing at the Boston Marathon. The problem was that I'd come away from Boston with a sore heel, which in Orange County became *a very painful heel*. Not only was I forced to drop out of that race, but I wasn't able to run again for several more weeks, spoiling my preparation for an Ironman triathlon I'd already paid for but wound up missing.

A part of me knew I was making a dumb decision even as I committed to it, but like other runners, "experts" sometimes allow emotion to overrule their reason, resulting in choices we later regret. Although perfect judgment is beyond our reach, we can learn from our missteps so we're less prone to repeating them. I'm happy to say that I make far fewer dumb decisions than I did when I was younger.

One thing that's helped me in this regard is a mental trick I call "asking for a friend." We all know this familiar phrase, which is typically uttered with a wink when we seek an answer to an awkward question. The friend we're asking for is almost always ourselves, and everyone knows it, but even so, the rhetorical fig leaf eases our embarrassment. I find a version of the same trick useful when I'm tempted to make a dumb decision. The twist is that, instead of seeking advice for a friend who's actually me, I pretend the person in my situation is someone else and I'm advising them.

It is a scientifically proven fact that people tend to make riskier choices for themselves than they would for someone else in situations involving physical safety (such as sitting next to a visibly sick passenger on an airplane or running a marathon with an injured foot) and in matters of the heart (like breaking curfew to extend a promising first date—or running a second, "rebound" marathon to salve the disappointment of a bad first one). The best way I know to overcome this inconsistency is to step outside myself and look at the decision in front of me objectively, as a friend might. It might seem a bit gimmicky, but with a little practice you're likely to find that "asking for a friend" works for you, too. ∎

© Ulf Bodin/gettyimages

Distance carried forward:

7 Monday 281

Where & When: **Distance:**
Comments:

8 Tuesday 282

Where & When: **Distance:**
Comments:

9 Wednesday 283

Where & When: **Distance:**
Comments:

10 Thursday 284

Where & When: **Distance:**
Comments:

11 Friday 285

Where & When: **Distance:**
Comments:

October

Saturday 12

286

Where & When: Distance:
Comments:

Sunday 13

287

Where & When: Distance:
Comments:

© Cavan Images/gettyimages

tip: Autumn is the best time of year to go after personal bests. The combination of summer fitness and cool fall temperatures is a recipe for performance breakthroughs.

Distance this week: Weight:

Distance carried forward:

14 Monday　　　　　　　　　　　　　　　　　　　　　　　288

Where & When:　　　　　　　　　　**Distance:**
Comments:

15 Tuesday　　　　　　　　　　　　　　　　　　　　　　289

Where & When:　　　　　　　　　　**Distance:**
Comments:

16 Wednesday　　　　　　　　　　　　　　　　　　　　290

Where & When:　　　　　　　　　　**Distance:**
Comments:

17 Thursday　　　　　　　　　　　　　　　　　　　　　291

Where & When:　　　　　　　　　　**Distance:**
Comments:

18 Friday　　　　　　　　　　　　　　　　　　　　　　　292

Where & When:　　　　　　　　　　**Distance:**
Comments:

October

Saturday 19

293

Where & When: Distance:
Comments:

Sunday 20

294

Where & When: Distance:
Comments:

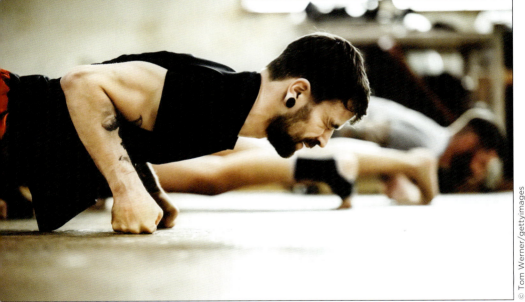

tip: Make a habit of doing something you don't enjoy *because* you don't enjoy it. Take cold showers, drink noni juice, or practice a strength exercise you particularly dislike. Such measures cultivate a mindset of embracing discomfort that will translate to the racecourse.

Distance this week: Weight:

Distance carried forward: _____

21 Monday 295

_____
_____

Where & When: _____ **Distance:** _____
Comments: _____

22 Tuesday 296

_____
_____

Where & When: _____ **Distance:** _____
Comments: _____

23 Wednesday 297

_____
_____

Where & When: _____ **Distance:** _____
Comments: _____

24 Thursday 298

_____
_____

Where & When: _____ **Distance:** _____
Comments: _____

25 Friday 299

_____
_____

Where & When: _____ **Distance:** _____
Comments: _____

October

Saturday 26

300

Where & When:　　　　　　　　　　　　　Distance:
Comments:

Sunday 27

301

Where & When:　　　　　　　　　　　　　Distance:
Comments:

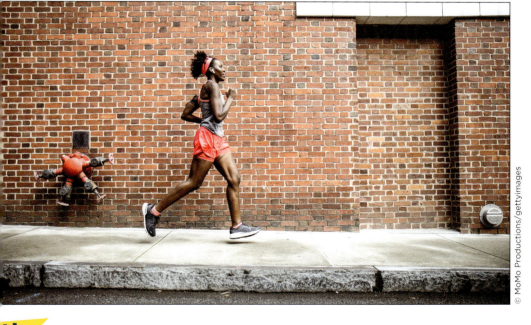

tip: Scientists analyzing data from more than fourteen thousand runners found that the fittest and fastest runners trained slower—relative to their ability—than other runners on their easy days. Beware the moderate-intensity rut!

Distance this week:　　　　　　　　　　　Weight:

Distance carried forward:

28 Monday 302

Where & When: **Distance:**
Comments:

29 Tuesday 303

Where & When: **Distance:**
Comments:

30 Wednesday 304

Where & When: **Distance:**
Comments:

31 Thursday 305

Where & When: **Distance:**
Comments:

1 Friday 306

Where & When: **Distance:**
Comments:

Oct/Nov

307

Saturday 2

Where & When: _____ Distance: _____
Comments: _____

308

Sunday 3

Where & When: _____ Distance: _____
Comments: _____

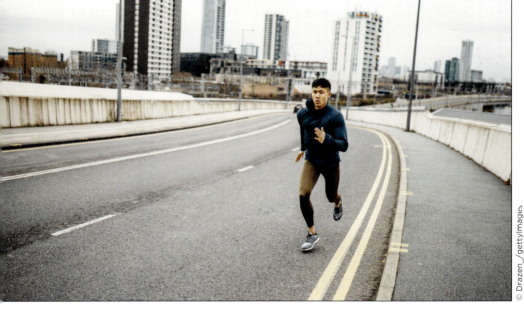

tip: Resist the temptation to "keep the momentum going" after a big race by continuing to train intensively. Give your body the break it needs. You'll be fitter for the next big race if you give some fitness away after this one.

Distance this week: _____ Weight: _____

November

SUNDAY	MONDAY	TUESDAY	WEDNESDAY	THURSDAY	FRIDAY	SATURDAY
					1	2
					● New Moon	
3	4	5	6	7	8	9
Daylight Saving Time ends (USA, Canada)		Election Day (USA)				◐ First Quarter
10	11	12	13	14	15	16
Remembrance Sunday (UK, Ireland)	Veterans Day (USA) Remembrance Day (Canada, UK, Ireland, Australia)				○ Full Moon	
17	18	19	20	21	22	23
						◑ Last Quarter
24	25	26	27	28	29	30
				Thanksgiving (USA)		St. Andrew's Day (UK)

tip: Consider choosing a power word or mantra to take into your next race—something that will give you just the reminder you need to get through difficult moments.

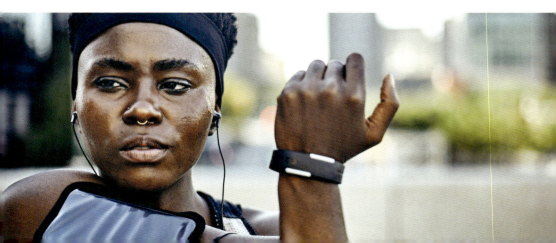

REMEMBER TO SAY THANK-YOU

I've always been an injury-prone runner. Tendon injuries in particular are my bane. Scientists have learned that specific gene variants related to collagen formation predispose certain athletes to tendon injuries. I'm willing to bet I have those genes. Three separate cases of tendinopathy—one in the knee, another in the Achilles, a third in the hip—have each kept me out of competition for more than a year.

The silver lining to my fragility is that it has heightened my appreciation for the gift of running. Each time I've come out the other side of an injury that I thought might end my running days permanently, I've felt immense gratitude. And although the initial rush of euphoria dims as my latest injury recedes into the past, it never goes away completely. I'm a more grateful runner in general than I would be if I hadn't gotten hurt so much.

The psychology at play here is quite normal. Losing something we love makes us more grateful once it's been restored. Even just the threat of loss can have this effect—in 2018, my friend Sarah underwent an operation to remove a tumor in her left thigh. Though technically benign, the growth was so large that her surgeon couldn't promise she would be able to return to running afterward. This would be bad news for any runner, but it was especially bad for Sarah because she ran professionally. On the advice of another friend, she ran alone in her favorite place the day before the operation. Running had never seemed more precious to her than it did in that solitary hour.

Less than two months later, still sporting stitches and a bandage, Sarah stood at the start of the Chicago Marathon, happy just to be there—a marked change from the year before, when she stood in the very same place thinking, *Why do I do this to myself?* Cold and wet conditions wrought havoc on the elite field in 2018, but Sarah's grateful mindset enabled her not only to survive the battle of attrition but finish sixth overall and first among Americans with a seven-second personal best.

"It had never really occurred to me that running was a choice," she told me later. "Only when the option to make that choice was threatened did I truly appreciate how much I actually did want to be out there running a marathon and hurting like hell."

You don't have to get injured or receive a scary medical diagnosis to run with gratitude. Studies have shown that people have more fun doing activities like running when they switch from a "have to" mindset to a grateful "get to" mindset. So, remember to say thank-you—to your body, to the road you tread, and to the air you breathe—in your next and every run. ∎

Distance carried forward:

4 Monday 309

Where & When: **Distance:**
Comments:

5 Tuesday 310

Where & When: **Distance:**
Comments:

6 Wednesday 311

Where & When: **Distance:**
Comments:

7 Thursday 312

Where & When: **Distance:**
Comments:

8 Friday 313

Where & When: **Distance:**
Comments:

November

314

Saturday 9

Where & When: Distance:
Comments:

315

Sunday 10

Where & When: Distance:
Comments:

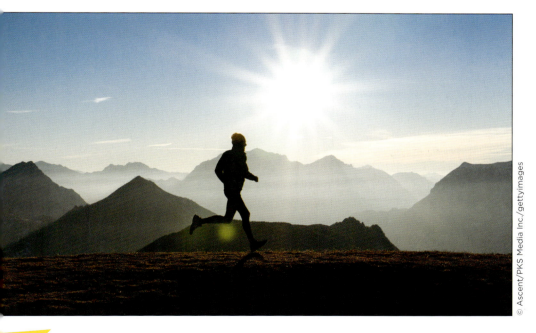

tip: Fall is windy season in many locations. Be sure to account for the effect of wind on pace and effort in your runs, just as you do with hills.

Distance this week: Weight:

Distance carried forward: _____

11 Monday   316

_____

Where & When: _____   **Distance:** _____
Comments: _____

12 Tuesday   317

_____

Where & When: _____   **Distance:** _____
Comments: _____

13 Wednesday   318

_____

Where & When: _____   **Distance:** _____
Comments: _____

14 Thursday   319

_____

Where & When: _____   **Distance:** _____
Comments: _____

15 Friday   320

_____

Where & When: _____   **Distance:** _____
Comments: _____

November

321   **Saturday 16**

Where & When: Distance:
Comments:

322   **Sunday 17**

Where & When: Distance:
Comments:

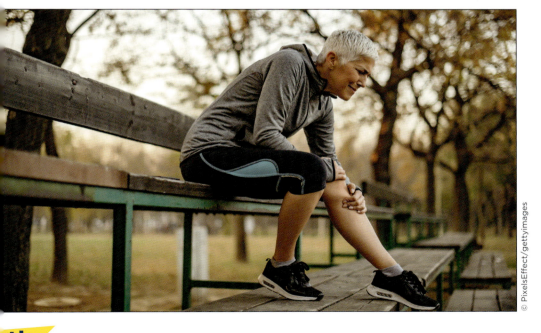

tip: Most major overuse injuries start off as minor sore spots. To prevent small problems from becoming big ones, react quickly to the emergence of sore spots by modifying your training appropriately, such as taking a day off or switching to cross-training.

Distance this week: Weight:

Distance carried forward:

18 Monday 323

Where & When: Distance:
Comments:

19 Tuesday 324

Where & When: Distance:
Comments:

20 Wednesday 325

Where & When: Distance:
Comments:

21 Thursday 326

Where & When: Distance:
Comments:

22 Friday 327

Where & When: Distance:
Comments:

November

Saturday 23

328

Where & When: Distance:
Comments:

Sunday 24

329

Where & When: Distance:
Comments:

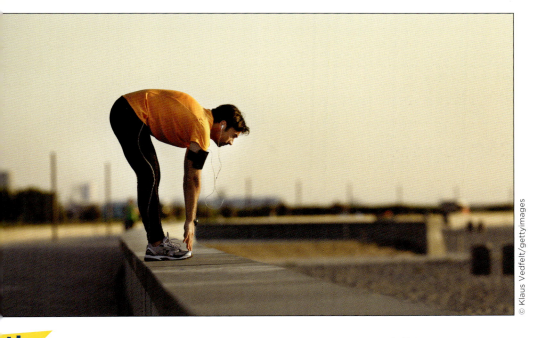

tip: A fun game you can play to improve your pacing skill is to set your device to autosplit every mile and guess your time before you check it.

Distance this week: Weight:

Distance carried forward:

25 Monday 330

Where & When: **Distance:**
Comments:

26 Tuesday 331

Where & When: **Distance:**
Comments:

27 Wednesday 332

Where & When: **Distance:**
Comments:

28 Thursday 333

Where & When: **Distance:**
Comments:

29 Friday 334

Where & When: **Distance:**
Comments:

Nov/Dec

335   **Saturday 30**

Where & When: Distance:

Comments:

336   **Sunday 1**

Where & When: Distance:

Comments:

© Heath Korvola/gettyimages

tip: With shorter, colder days comes less sun exposure, lower vitamin D levels, and sluggishness for many runners. This might be a good time to have your vitamin D checked or take a supplement.

Distance this week: Weight:

December

SUNDAY	MONDAY	TUESDAY	WEDNESDAY	THURSDAY	FRIDAY	SATURDAY
1 ● New Moon	2	3	4	5	6	7
8 ◐ First Quarter	9	10 Human Rights Day	11	12	13	14
15 ○ Full Moon	16	17	18	19	20	21 Winter Solstice
22 ◑ Last Quarter	23	24 Christmas Eve	25 Christmas Day Hanukkah (begins at sundown)	26 Kwanzaa begins (USA) Boxing Day (Canada, NZ, UK, Australia) St. Stephen's Day (Ireland) Proclamation Day (Australia—SA)	27	28
29	30 ● New Moon	31				

tip: A lot of runners conflate rest and recovery. Rest is simply not exercising, whereas recovery is the process of overcoming fatigue. Although recovery is the purpose of rest, you can also recover by doing less exercise than normal rather than none at all.

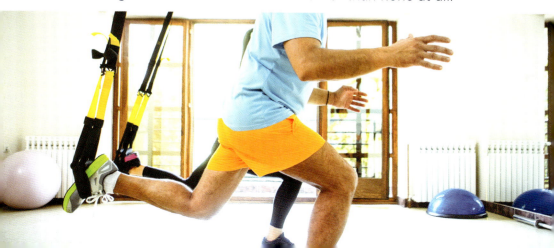

I AM A RUNNER

I have a confession to make. In preceding essays, I've written about my running in the present tense, implying that I have an ongoing running habit. The truth is that I haven't run in two years, not because I don't want to but because I can't. Or, more accurately, I could run, but it would make me very ill.

I am one of those who got sick with the coronavirus and never fully recovered. "Long COVID," as it has come to be known, is a mysterious chronic illness characterized by fatigue, brain fog, shortness of breath, and—get this—exercise intolerance. When I first developed these and other symptoms (nerve pain, insomnia, the list goes on), I kept running for a while, but every step was a struggle. Then I read about post-exertional malaise, a phenomenon first observed in people with chronic fatigue syndrome whereby physical exertion is followed by a delayed worsening of symptoms. The word "malaise" aptly described how I felt most of the time. So, I decided to pull the plug on my running entirely.

I did not, however, divorce myself from the sport, which, by choice and by necessity, has remained a big part of my life. As a running coach, author, and business owner, I spend a good chunk of each day thinking about running and interacting with runners. As my own training receded further into the past, though, there came a point where I began to feel self-conscious about calling myself a runner—so uncomfortable, in fact, that I chose to stop using the present tense in reference to my running. "I love eating pizza after long runs" became "I used to love eating pizza after long runs."

It was hard at first, but I figured it would get easier with time. It didn't. Because I still feel like a runner. When I hustle to cross a busy street, my body falls right back into those old, familiar rhythms. I still think like a runner, my mind chock-full of knowledge and memories that are as much a part of me as they ever were. And I still love running, as much as any runner. The only thing that's different, frankly, is that I can't actually run anymore. But that could change! For all of these reasons, I've gone back to the present tense, and once again proudly declare that I am a runner. ■

© Gilaxia/gettyimages

Distance carried forward:

2 Monday 337

Where & When: **Distance:**
Comments:

3 Tuesday 338

Where & When: **Distance:**
Comments:

4 Wednesday 339

Where & When: **Distance:**
Comments:

5 Thursday 340

Where & When: **Distance:**
Comments:

6 Friday 341

Where & When: **Distance:**
Comments:

December

342

Saturday 7

Where & When: Distance:
Comments:

343

Sunday 8

Where & When: Distance:
Comments:

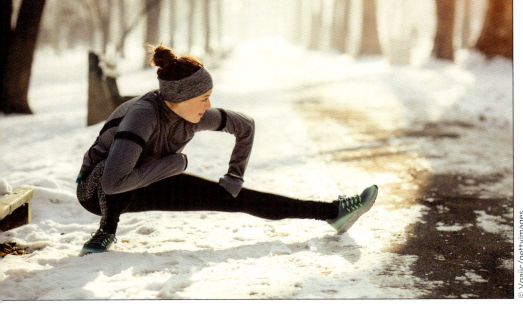

© Vgajic/gettyimages

tip: Pain does not always equal injury: It's both normal and acceptable to experience some pain during periods of intensive training. The thing to avoid is pain that worsens over the course of a run or from one run to the next.

Distance this week: Weight:

Distance carried forward:

9 Monday 344

Where & When: **Distance:**
Comments:

10 Tuesday 345

Where & When: **Distance:**
Comments:

11 Wednesday 346

Where & When: **Distance:**
Comments:

12 Thursday 347

Where & When: **Distance:**
Comments:

13 Friday 348

Where & When: **Distance:**
Comments:

December

Saturday 14

349

Where & When: Distance:
Comments:

Sunday 15

350

Where & When: Distance:
Comments:

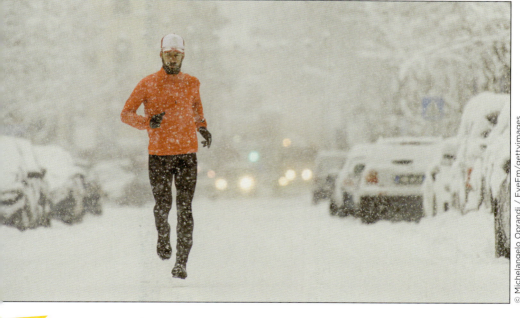

tip: While endurance training strengthens the immune system overall, bigger individual workouts temporarily suppress immune function, opening the door to infection. Be mindful and take appropriate precautions, especially during winter virus season.

Distance this week: Weight:

Distance carried forward: _____

16 Monday　　　　　　　　　　　　　　　　　　　　　35

_____
_____

Where & When: _____　　**Distance:** _____
Comments: _____

17 Tuesday　　　　　　　　　　　　　　　　　　　　352

_____
_____

Where & When: _____　　**Distance:** _____
Comments: _____

18 Wednesday　　　　　　　　　　　　　　　　　　　35:

_____
_____

Where & When: _____　　**Distance:** _____
Comments: _____

19 Thursday　　　　　　　　　　　　　　　　　　　354

_____
_____

Where & When: _____　　**Distance:** _____
Comments: _____

20 Friday　　　　　　　　　　　　　　　　　　　　355

_____
_____

Where & When: _____　　**Distance:** _____
Comments: _____

December

356   **Saturday 21**

Where & When: Distance:
Comments:

357   **Sunday 22**

Where & When: Distance:
Comments:

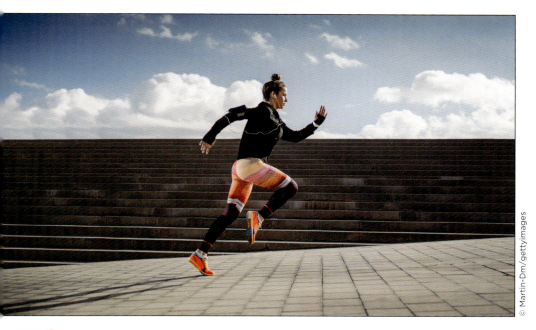

© Martin-Dm/gettyimages

tip: One of the most common mistakes runners make when tapering for races is cutting back too much on high intensity. Runners race better when the pre-race taper period includes judicious amounts of fast running.

Distance this week: Weight:

Distance carried forward:

23 Monday 358

Where & When: **Distance:**
Comments:

24 Tuesday 359

Where & When: **Distance:**
Comments:

25 Wednesday 360

Where & When: **Distance:**
Comments:

26 Thursday 361

Where & When: **Distance:**
Comments:

27 Friday 362

Where & When: **Distance:**
Comments:

December

Saturday 28

363

Where & When: Distance:
Comments:

Sunday 29

364

Where & When: Distance:
Comments:

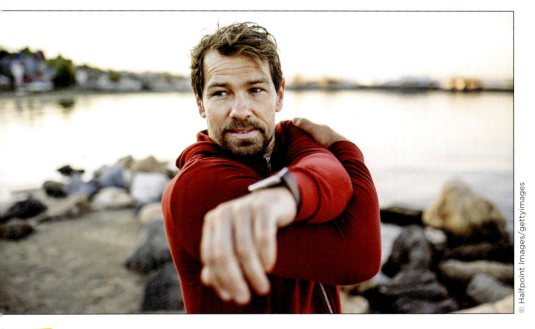

tip: You can't stop negative thoughts from happening during tough moments in workouts and races. What you can do is be prepared and have a plan for dealing with them. What's your plan?

Distance this week: Weight:

Distance carried forward:

30 Monday 365

Where & When: **Distance:**
Comments:

31 Tuesday 366

Where & When: **Distance:**
Comments:

1 Wednesday

Where & When: **Distance:**
Comments:

2 Thursday

Where & When: **Distance:**
Comments:

3 Friday

Where & When: **Distance:**
Comments:

Dec/Jan 2025

Saturday 4

Where & When: Distance:
Comments:

Sunday 5

Where & When: Distance:
Comments:

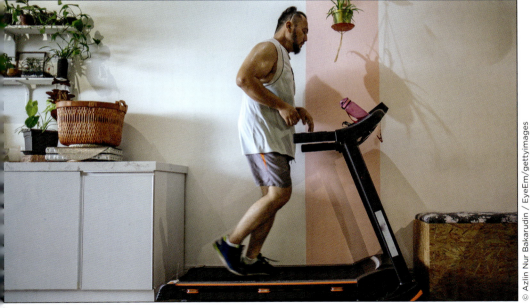

tip: In February 2000, Christine Clark won the U.S. Olympic Trials Women's Marathon having trained entirely on a treadmill over the winter in Anchorage, Alaska. Never doubt the effectiveness of indoor running!

Distance this week: Weight:

Twelve Months of Running

	Jan. 1	Jan. 8	Jan. 15	Jan. 22	Jan. 29	Feb. 5	Feb. 12	Feb. 19	Feb. 26	March 4	March 11	March 18	March 25

To create a cumulative bar graph of weekly mileage, apply an appropriate scale at the left-hand margin. Then fill in the bar for each week of running.

	Apr. 1	Apr. 8	Apr. 15	Apr. 22	Apr. 29	May 6	May 13	May 20	May 27	June 3	June 10	June 17	June 24

To create a cumulative bar graph of weekly mileage, apply an appropriate scale at the left-hand margin. Then fill in the bar for each week of running.

	July 1	July 8	July 15	July 22	July 29	Aug. 5	Aug. 12	Aug. 19	Aug. 26	Sept. 2	Sept. 9	Sept. 16	Sept. 23	Sept. 30

To create a cumulative bar graph of weekly mileage, apply an appropriate scale at the left-hand margin. Then fill in the bar for each week of running.

	Oct. 7	Oct. 14	Oct. 21	Oct. 28	Nov. 4	Nov. 11	Nov. 18	Nov. 25	Dec. 2	Dec. 9	Dec. 16	Dec. 23	Dec. 30

A Record of Races

Date	Place	Distance	Time	Pace	Comments & Excuses

A Record of Races

Date	Place	Distance	Time	Pace	Comments & Excuses

RACING

Pace is crucial. And you won't magically find it on race day. If you've resisted using a stopwatch or a heart monitor in your workouts, training for a 10K race is the perfect opportunity to abandon those prejudices.

10K

Warm up? Yes, even a slow half-mile run before the race is likely to improve your performance, not fatigue you. Remember that a 10K event is too short to grant you a sufficient warm-up during the race.

Divide the race into three equal segments and start slower than you want. Don't reach your race pace until the second segment. Push on the third. But your times between these three segments shouldn't vary by more than 10 percent.

Half Marathon

If you're running a half-marathon as preparation for a marathon, cut your weekly long run to no more than 12 miles and raise the pace.

Every week should include three types of workouts: speed drills, tempo runs, and your long run. Speed drills make you faster. Tempo runs raise your lactate threshold, which will help you maintain a racing pace in the second half of the event. And your weekly long run increases endurance. Toss in some cross-training when time allows.

Don't be shaken by early mistakes. If you go out too fast, for example, simply dial back as soon as you recognize your error. It's a long race and there's plenty of time to recover from just about any kind of blunder.

RACING

Marathon

No one masters the marathon. Anything can happen on its long tortuous course, which is why it is such a seductive and exciting event. It's in your interest to arrive at the starting line with this humility.

Seek support. Train with a partner or a running group. Get your loved ones to cheer you on at the race. Raise money for a cause. The road to the marathon can be long and lonely. Let others help you get there.

Believe it or not, it's better to undertrain than to overtrain. What you haven't developed by race day can sometimes be overcome with adrenaline and desire. For an overtrained runner, the race is over before it starts.

Triathlon

Get used to crowding. In open water where visibility is often poor, contact with other swimmers is inevitable. On bicycles it can be dangerous. Patience pays. Fighting through a pack of competitors wastes energy and can throw your race into jeopardy. Relax. Your opportunity to pass will come.

Rehearse transitions. Without specific training, it takes bicycling legs longer to reach their running stride than many athletes realize. Pulling dry socks onto wet feet can be an ordeal. Fussing with uncooperative equipment squanders time.

Your weakest event deserves the greatest amount of training effort. Sorry, it's true. Most triathletes use their best event to make up time. The better strategy is not to lose time in your weak event.

JANUARY 2025

FEBRUARY 2025

MARCH 2025

APRIL 2025

MAY 2025

JUNE 2025

JULY 2025

AUGUST 2025

SEPTEMBER 2025

OCTOBER 2025

NOVEMBER 2025

DECEMBER 2025